Holding Fast

Increasing pressure on caregiving organizations to serve more people with fewer resources means that epidemics of burnout, high staff turnover, dissatisfaction and internal conflict often appear inevitable. *Holding Fast* focuses on the particular stress of caregiving work, its influences on the people and organizations who do that work, and what they can do about it.

Illustrated by case studies based on extensive research in schools, hospitals, social work agencies, healthcare centres and religious institutions, *Holding Fast* identifies the problems faced by caregiving organizations, and outlines appropriate strategies for tackling these to create a resilient, effective organization. The book is divided into clear sections covering:

- an introduction to the nature of caregiving organizations
- the disturbances that can occur within them
- the skills required to effectively lead them.

Holding Fast offers a portrait of how organizations become or are prevented from becoming systems of caregiving. It will help leaders of caregiving organizations and their staff gain a better understanding of the difficulties encountered by their organizations, leading to improved management and practice.

William A. Kahn is Associate Professor in the Department of Organizational Behavior at Boston University's School of Management, where he teaches courses on leadership and organizational change to MBA students and executives.

Holding Fast

The Struggle to Create Resilient Caregiving Organizations

William A. Kahn

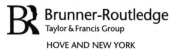

Brunner-Routledge
Taylor & Francis Group
HOVE AND NEW YORK

First published 2005 by Brunner-Routledge
27 Church Road, Hove, East Sussex, BN3 2FA

Simultaneously published in the USA and Canada
by Brunner-Routledge
270 Madison Avenue, New York, NY 10016

Brunner-Routledge is an imprint of the Taylor & Francis Group

Typeset in Times by RefineCatch Ltd, Bungay, Suffolk
Printed and bound in Great Britain by
TJ International, Padstow, Cornwall
Paperback cover design by Hybert Design

British Library Cataloguing in Publication Data
A catalogue record for this book is available from the British Library

Library of Congress Cataloging-in-Publication Data
Kahn, William A., 1959–
   Holding fast: the struggle to create resilient caregiving
organizations / William A. Kahn.
       p.   cm.
Includes bibliographical references and index.
   ISBN 1-58391-936-8 (hardback : alk. paper) –
ISBN 1-58391-937-6 (pbk. : alk. paper)
   1. Human services.   2. Human services personnel – job
stress.   3. Caregivers – job stress.   4. Human services –
Management.   5. Organizational effectiveness.   6. Counselor and
client.   I. Title.
HV40.K265 2004
361'.0068'3 – dc22   2004013760

ISBN 1-58391-936-8 (Hbk)
ISBN 1-58391-937-6 (Pbk)

To Dana, for holding fast and holding well

Contents

Preface

In my years of working with organizations as a researcher and consultant I have found myself drawn to certain kinds of places. Schools, hospitals, social service agencies, mental health centers, residential treatment centers, churches and synagogues, daycare and geriatric centers – we have sought each other out, it seems, for these places comprise much of my work. These organizations are of a type. They contain similar issues that present themselves for resolution. These include seeming epidemics of stress and burnout, teams in disarray, gulfs between the front lines and the back offices, conflicts within and between groups and departments. It is possible, of course, that these issues present themselves because I look for them and the organizations oblige, used as they are to providing for the needs of others. It is also possible that these organizations share nothing more than my interest, rather than some classification that renders them alike in some meaningful way.

I have grown increasingly convinced, however, that these organizations share a common denominator. They are *caregiving organizations*, a class that subsumes the traditional category of "human service" or "helping" organizations. Caregiving organizations are those whose members provide care to people who seek healing, growth, ministry, learning or support of one kind or another. It is in the nature of the caregiving task that certain issues are triggered, for the organizations and their members; it is in the nature of the caregiving work that questions are posed that must be resolved if that work is to be ultimately effective.

I decided to take seriously this idea that there is such a thing as a caregiving organization, which manifests itself across various sectors that include education, healthcare, ministry, social services, residential treatment, and psychiatric facilities. Each of these sectors, of course, has its own significant literature and those literatures offer a great many useful theoretical frameworks and practical ideas. There is much to be gained, however, from examining these organizations *as* caregiving organizations, that is, as institutions whose members bring resources to bear on healing, ministering to, growing, and in other ways caring for those who approach them bearing needs, anxieties, and other aspects of their humanity. This transaction is or ought to be at the core of the caregiving organization, regardless of its sector. By examining that core we can learn about the essential nature of these organizations. We can learn what makes them resilient in the face of the ongoing stress of their caregiving tasks.

Resilient organizations, like individuals, have the capacity to absorb stress and difficult emotions without being so harmed that they cannot function effectively. They may sway and bend under the weight of what they absorb but they do not break; they maintain the capacity to right themselves. My study of caregiving organizations has shown me that resilience may be a property of the collective – that organizations and their units may create cultures of resilience that sustain themselves through the loss of individual members. In resilient cultures, members have figured out how to learn and grow in the midst of difficult, sometimes painful environments; they have learned to remain connected to rather than disconnected from one another and careseekers. This is not a simple proposition, and many caregiving organizations struggle to make it true.

I ground this book in both theory and actual case studies of caregiving organizations as they struggle for resilience and effectiveness. The theoretical concepts reflect various disciplines that include organizational behavior and management, group and intergroup relations theory, psychodynamic and clinical psychology. The case studies are from action research that I have conducted over the past 15 years with schools, hospitals, social work agencies, healthcare units, residential treatment centers, and religious institutions. These organizations are, of course, different. They are also alike in important ways that often go unacknowledged. Each case study illustrates the particular context of a particular organization and its sector. Collectively, they offer a portrait of how organizations become, or are prevented from becoming, resilient systems of caregiving.

Acknowledgements

This book owes its existence to the members and leaders of the various caregiving organizations who participated in the action research and consultation projects that provided so much of the material contained here. They allowed me, and themselves, to engage in extended, often difficult examinations of their practices, and did their best to change familiar but dysfunctional habits of thought and action. They struggled well. I am indebted to their allowing me to learn from their struggles.

I am indebted as well to several individuals whose intellectual companionship and personal support were invaluable, not simply during the writing of this book but in the years that led me toward this work. Joe Allen, David Berg, and Linda Powell have each provided both safe harbor and intellectual challenge when I found myself tossed about by some wave or other of uncertainty or frustration. Working with caregiving organizations is often quite draining, in ways which I sometimes forget when in the midst of a project. Each of these colleagues and friends have found occasion to remind me of this, and in doing so held me until I regained equilibrium. I also appreciate the steady support of the Brookline Circle, whose members include Lee Bolman, Dave Brown, Tim Hall, Todd Jick, Phil Mirvis, and Barry Oshry.

I also gratefully acknowledge permission to reproduce quotations from the following works: *Containing Anxiety in Institutions, Volume 1* by Isabel Menzies Lyth, with permission from Free Association Books Ltd, copyright © 1988; *Dependence* by Albert Memmi, copyright © 1984 by Beacon Press, translated by Philip A. Facey from La Dependence © Editions Gallimard, 1979 and reprinted by permission of Beacon Press, Boston; *From Dependence to Autonomy* by Eric E. Miller, with permission from Free Association Books Ltd, copyright © 1993; *Generation to Generation* by Edwin H. Friedman with permission from The Guilford Press, copyright © 1995; *Strengthening Family Resilience* by Froma Walsh with permission from The Guilford Press, copyright © 1998; *The Personality of the Organization* by Lionel Stapley, with permission from Free Association Books Ltd, copyright © 1996; *The Unconscious at Work*, edited by Anton Obholzer and Vega Zagier Roberts, with permission from Routledge, copyright © 1994; *The Wisdom of the Ego* by George E. Vaillant, Cambridge, MA: Harvard University Press, copyright © 1993 by the President and Fellows of Harvard College; *Thinking About Institutions: Milieux and Madness* by R. D. Hinshelwood with permission from Jessica Kingsley Publishers, Copyright © 2001 R. D. Hinshelwood.

A note on confidentiality

The case illustrations used in this book have been drawn from action research and consultation with specific caregiving organizations. All names are fictitious and identifying details have been altered to preserve the anonymity of those involved.

Part I

The nature of caregiving organizations

Caregiving organizations are marked by the essential gesture of some people caring for others. Such caring is manifested differently in different settings. In schools, it appears in the context of teachers helping students learn, about themselves and their worlds. In hospitals and other heathcare institutions, it appears as physicians, nurses, and specialists diagnosing and treating patients who seek healing. In residential treatment centers, caring appears in the therapeutic, often difficult interactions between staff and clients. In social service agencies, it appears in the context of social workers helping clients learn to navigate the shoals of their lives. In churches and synagogues, it appears in the relations between clergy and the congregants who seek meaning, grace, and peacefulness. Each of these settings may differ, in terms of the population it serves and how it does so. Yet each setting shares with one another an essential gesture: the creation of relationships between those who provide and those who seek some form of care, in the form of learning, healing, or growing in some fashion or another. That gesture lies at the heart of the caregiving organization.

The relationship between caregivers and careseekers holds the key that unlocks a complex understanding of caregiving organizations, be they schools, hospitals, churches, social service agencies, nursing homes, and the like. That relationship brings careseekers into the organization in certain ways. It places certain demands and requirements upon individual caregivers, and more generally, upon the caregiving organization. Individuals and organizations both react in certain ways, which vary from useful to dysfunctional, from resilient to disturbed, with direct implications for the organization's ability to meet the needs of careseekers and members alike. Caregiving relationships thus reverberate throughout the larger systems in which they are embedded, which react in ways that reverberate back to those relationships, creating an enclosed feedback loop that may be more, or less, healthy for all involved.

Part 1 contains four chapters that together offer a theoretical framework for understanding these dynamics and the underlying nature of caregiving organizations. Chapter 1 describes the nature of the relationship between caregivers and careseekers and its implications for the caregiving organization more generally. Chapter 2 focuses on the different types of strains that press upon caregivers and other caregiving organization members. Chapter 3 describes the nature of resilient caregiving organizations, whose members create cultures and practices that enable them to live and work well with the strains presented earlier. Chapter 4 articulates the nature of caregiving organizations that prove to be not resilient but disturbed in some fashion by the strain of caregiving work. The theoretical framework and concepts embedded in these chapters offer a foundation for later chapters, focusing on the application of concepts to specific caregiving organizations.

Chapter 1

Caregiving organizations defined

Karen sits at her desk, trying to find the energy to complete her case notes. She lifts her cup of coffee then wearily puts it down upon discovering it has grown cold. It is the end of a typically bruising day. She visited four families in different parts of the city that morning. Each had been reported for a potential violation of the rules governing foster parenting. They were the usual visits. One woman began sobbing within a few minutes of Karen's arrival, hysterical because her husband had disappeared for four days and returned drunk. Another spent the entire visit trying to get Karen to increase her payments, while ignoring completely the small boy complaining tearfully of an ache in his side. Karen's last visit that morning was with a teenage girl who spoke little but flinched whenever the foster father walked near her. Karen returned to the office for an afternoon meeting about a new policy directive. She knew the policy made little sense, and tried to say so, but her supervisor said they had no choice and had to go ahead with it. Karen and the other social workers rolled their eyes. Later, she looked for the super-visor to help her think about the teenage girl at the last visit but found that she was in meetings for the rest of the day with the executive director and other administrators. The other senior social workers were too busy as well, on the phone or at court or with families. It has been like this for a while, people too busy to talk with one another. The agency has lost people – the usual turnover – and with the current job market they have been unable to replace social workers. The supervisor is the third person to hold the position in the last 18 months. The executive director spends time with the board, trying to drum up support and funding for new programs. It is tough going. He is overwhelmed by the work of trying to keep the agency afloat. Karen slumps down in her chair, suddenly aware of just how tired she is.

This scene is not unique to social workers or to this agency. With the circumstances and contexts changed slightly, Karen could just as easily be a teacher, nurse, minister, therapist, or childcare worker. Her agency could just as easily be a school, hospital, church, counseling center, or residential treatment facility. Each of these is a *caregiving organization* – an institution whose members directly provide for people who seek healing, growth, ministry, learning or support of one kind or another. What is unique to these organizations is how the work itself puts a special stress on individuals. This is what gets people and organizations in trouble, causing typical problems like burnout and turnover, lack of teamwork, and uneasy relations between administrators and direct caregivers. This book focuses on the particular stress of caregiving work, its influences on the people and organizations who do that work, and what they can do about it.

Caregiving organizations are in the business of responding to people's needs. Schools take in youths who need to learn what they do not know and deal with the needs of anxious parents and communities. Hospitals respond to patients' needs for healing. Churches and synagogues work with people's needs to understand and cope with the events of their lives. Counseling centers work with people to help with mental illness or emotional distress. Social service agencies help people get on track with their lives in the face of difficult circumstances. Residential schools and treatment centers take in people who need healthy relationships and support. All of these needs are of a type: they involve people's emotions and anxieties. People do not approach these organizations simply to buy products, like at retail stores, or be serviced, like at hotels, or entertained, like at theaters. People become patients or clients of these organizations because they need help or need to grow, often within circumstances that make them frightened or confused or anxious. This very fact – that people bring their human needs into their transactions with members of these organizations – fundamentally shapes what occurs in those organizations, with clients and among members themselves. Also, it distinguishes these organizations from others, like banks or hotels, which also serve to meet people's needs. Such service organizations do not routinely work with the anxiety and distress that often accompany people's experiences in caregiving organizations. Nor are they routinely confronted with the full ranges of emotions that often accompany people's difficult, joyous, enraging, powerful journeys toward growth, healing, and learning.

Describing an institution as a caregiving organization seems, at first glance, redundant with current classifications. There are human service organizations, which provide social and health services to individuals in various stages of need and disrepair. There are people who work in the so-called helping professions; they too are often located in human service organizations. And there are the sectors themselves: education, religion, healthcare, social services, residential treatment, psychiatry, geriatrics, and the like. Each of these has associated with it various types of organization by which clients are served. So why introduce yet another category, that of the caregiving organization?

The answer lies in the nature of the primary technology by which these organizations work. Caregiving organizations, in their various manifestations, bring together one group of people who need some form of care with another group of people, who provide for such care. They do so through the vehicle of their own direct relationships with careseekers. It is this set of conditions – one group directly caring for another, through the technology of personal relationships – that defines the caregiving organization, as it goes about its primary task.

Primary tasks

The primary task of an organization is that which it must perform in order to survive (Rice 1958). This is a normative definition, focusing on what people ought to do given the purposes for which they have come together. Systems or sub-systems have at any given time tasks which they were created to perform (Rice 1958). Primary tasks are thus tasks that people in an organization ought to pursue, as defined by a superordinate authority (Miller 1993). They are crucial for an institution's survival. In some instances, this is relatively straightforward. The primary tasks of manufacturing corporations are to make a profit by making and selling goods. In other instances, there are multiple tasks competing for primacy. Lyth (1988) offers the example of a teaching hospital, in which the primary task of caring for patients at times yields to that of training medical and nursing students. Caregiving organizations often contain multiple tasks, which compete for legitimacy. Such competition may obscure the reality that unless the needs of careseekers are served, the caregiving organization will not, in the long run, survive.

Different caregiving organizations have different primary tasks. Schools exist to teach people what they do not know. Hospitals strive to heal the sick. Residential centers exist by providing ongoing treatment across a variety of activities. Churches and synagogues exist by ministering to spiritual needs through rituals, texts, and dialogue. Social service agencies exist by meeting the needs of community members through the accrual and disbursement of resources. Nursing homes exist by meeting the end-of-life needs of residents and family members. Daycare centers exist by creating safe, engaging activities for growing, learning children. Psychiatric institutions exist by containing or improving, through chemical and therapeutic interventions, the mental illness of their patients. Each of these tasks is crucial to the survival of these organizations; and each task seems quite different from the other.

Beneath the surface, however, the primary tasks of caregiving organizations depend, invariably, on much the same process: the effective providing and receiving of care. The process of caring for others is, at its heart, not simply a technical matter. It is not simply the surgeon's technique, the lesson plan of the teacher facing a new class, the psychiatrist's diagnosis of a schizophrenic patient. It is not simply the flow of nurses across their shift, the breaking up of a fight at a daycare center, the applying for a grant to fund a new program for the homeless, the minister's sermon after a difficult week in her community. Caregiving involves all of these, and countless other technical actions like them. But at its heart, the essential technology by which the organization performs its task is that of the *relationships* between caregivers – nurses, teachers, therapists, ministers, social workers, physicians, and the like – and those who need their help.

The point of this book is to examine these various organizations *as* caregiving organizations, as one might examine people's underlying skeletal structures to better understand their movements, regardless of body size and type. The premise here is that such an analysis will illuminate issues that occur in these organizations because of the caregiving nature of their work. Indeed, the premise is that a diagnosis of how these various organizations function as caregiving institutions will illuminate their true natures, and in turn the true sources of any dysfunction they maintain. In this chapter, I begin the process of illuminating the essential nature of caregiving organizations, across body size and type.

The primacy of relationships

People best grow, heal, and learn in the context of meaningful relationships. Students learn best in relation with caring teachers. Patients heal best when they experience themselves as cared for by nurses, therapists, and physicians. Children and adults assume more responsibility for their recovery from abuse, addiction, and neglect when they feel seen, valued, and cared for by social workers and other caregivers. Worshippers feel more spiritually ministered to in relation with religious workers they experience as valuing and caring. Such relationships are a primary determinant of how well needs for support, knowledge, healing, and growth are met. It is at the point of contact between careseekers and caregivers that the former experience themselves as meaningfully taken in (or not) and cared for (or not) by caregiving institutions.

The emphasis here on such relationships is based on the premise that growth, healing, and learning often involves risk and vulnerability for people. Students often feel fearful about showing themselves as unable to master new skills and material, anxious about how they fit in with others, and uncertain about whom they are becoming. Sick patients struggle with fears about pain, diminished capacities, and death. The indigent, abused, and neglected may be sad, angry, or hopeless. Those seeking spiritual comfort may feel powerless and uncertain in the face of mortality and existential questions about meaning. These people bring and entrust their selves, and their anxieties, to caregiving organizations. For any of them to move ahead in the face of their anxieties requires, often enough, a safe-enough relationship with others they experience as caring.

Without that sense of safety, it is difficult for people to move toward engaging their own growth and development. Such active engagement is crucial (Mayeroff 1971; Memmi 1974; Rogers 1958). Students must take risks, launching themselves toward discovery of what they do not know; they must raise their hands and display curiosity and probe further, and in doing so, risk censure. Patients must take up the cause of their own healing. While bodies might well heal of their own accord – the broken leg mends, scar tissue covers a wound – the creation of meaningful relationships hastens the healing of people's other, less observable, parts which may also be wounded and lay hurting. Careseekers who are in need of social services must themselves seek out those services, and must use them properly and consistently, if they are to help themselves out of their difficult circumstances. Congregants troubled by spiritual dilemmas must seek, and question, and involve themselves in conversation and ritual until they have reached some insight and meaning that offers them satisfaction. Each of these represents careseekers venturing forth to engage their journeys toward health, growth, and learning. Each represents relationships with caregivers who offer careseekers a sense of security, a place to which they can return should they become momentarily overwhelmed.

This pattern is rooted in the earliest process of people moving toward their own growth and development: childhood. Mary Ainsworth developed the idea, based on attachment theory (Bowlby 1980), of a *secure base* to explain how children were able to move away from their caregivers, usually mothers (Ainsworth 1967). Attachment theory focuses on how relationships between children and attachment figures facilitate or undermine children feeling secure. Children who receive effective caregiving engage in exploratory behaviors, consisting of movements away from attachment figures in order to investigate surroundings, gain knowledge and skills, and cope with or control the environment (Ainsworth 1990). Secure base relations enable children to engage in unworried explorations, trusting their parents/attachment figures to come to their aid should difficulties arise (Ainsworth 1967). Other children are less able to engage in unworried exploration. Their explorations tend to be anxious, frustrated, or inhibited (Heard 1982). Attachment figures create secure base relations when they act as effective caregivers, consistently performing behaviors that lead their children to feel secure and able to explore.

While the secure base concept was developed in relation to children and their attachment figures, it applies to adult relations as well (Ainsworth 1990; Weiss 1982). The search for a secure base occurs throughout the life cycle, especially in emergencies. Adults as well as children seek out familiar individuals willing and able to offer aid in emergencies (Bowlby 1988). The secure base concept offers a particularly useful way to conceptualize what people need when they experience themselves, as they will at various moments in their growth, as lost, confused, frightened, anxious, or threatened.

The relationship between caregiver and careseeker echoes, sometimes faintly and other times loudly, the dynamics of secure base relations. A student is about to take an exam about which he is quite anxious. A recovering drug addict wavers in the face of a difficult personal situation. A surgical patient is having difficulty managing the pain medication. A congregant's faith wavers in the face of a tragic accident to a family member. An abused youth at a residential treatment center feels upset at yet another broken promise from his mother and feels enraged at his housemates. In each of these situations, the careseeker experiences anxiety, perhaps to the point of being overwhelmed. A choice point presents itself: does the careseeker retreat in the face of that anxiety, that is, move away from rather than toward the path of growth, healing, and learning? Does the student avoid or give up on the test, the addict take drugs, the patient take too much or too little medication, the congregant leave the congregation, the youth hurt his housemates? Or does the careseeker seek out someone – teacher, counselor, nurse, clergy, therapist – with whom there is a trusting, caring relationship, one that provides the support necessary to keep on the path?

Such choice points are only possible, of course, to the extent that caregivers have created trusting relationships through repeated acts of caregiving. In doing so, they create themselves as secure bases, to which others may momentarily repair when they find themselves startled, temporarily overwhelmed by anxiety. Metaphorically, careseekers at times find themselves in deep waters, as they go about facing what they have not faced before in their selves or in their environments. They may suddenly discover that they are not on safe ground as they once were. They may flounder and panic, as people do when waves are too high or currents too strong and they are unsure of their abilities to remain afloat. When they have caregivers in whom they trust, however, they are tethered. The caregivers support them, their weight back and feet digging into the shore, as they hold lifelines connected to those who have waded out into what is for them uncharted waters. Careseekers are held fast.

The nature of caregiving

Such tethering begins with acts of caregiving. These appear different in different institutions. In a school, a teacher sits with a struggling student during recess and patiently works with him on a mathematics concept. In a hospital, a physician huddles with a nurse before walking over to a patient and her family and discussing the effects of the latest treatment and next steps. In a geriatric home, a nursing aide meets with a group of patients to plan a holiday party. In a social service agency, a social worker treats a group of youths to ice-cream as they talk about their summer plans. Any such act offers the grounds for caregiving interactions. What is crucial is the underlying, essential gesture of caring: an attention to the person of the other in ways that leave them feeling valued.

In practice this is a constant series of calibrations. Caregivers move toward others by inquiring into their experiences, listening attentively, and providing resources. They move away from them as well, giving them the space to practice, to fail, to draw on and develop their own resources. Effective caregivers neither intrude nor abandon, i.e., are neither too unresponsive (when others seek proximity or help) nor overactive and impinging (when others need to explore and operate on their own). Instead, they remain emotionally present, ready to come to aid should the need arise (Kahn 1992, 1998). They remain at a safe distance, from which they safely guide others while enabling them to rely on and develop their selves. If one were to look closely beneath the acts that enable careseekers to grow, heal, and learn, across a variety of institutions they join for that purpose, one would see relationships in which caregivers are present, and safely distant, simultaneously. These relationships make it more likely that students will master difficult material, patients will take on difficult therapies, addicts will face their own addictions, youth will look at rather than act out their destructive impulses, and congregants will examine their moral behaviors. They will do so because they are both in relation to others who safeguard them, and at the same time, they are autonomous.

Consider the alternatives. A nurse comes over to the bedside of a patient who has been ringing her intermittently, complaining that his pain medication does not work. She glances at his chart, tells him the dosage looks fine, and walks away, telling a colleague that she's looking forward to "not dealing with the gall-bladder in room four" once her shift ends. A teacher routinely sends a student who becomes unusually troublesome whenever there is a grammar test to the headmaster for discipline. A social worker takes days to answer phone calls, telling her supervisor that she does not want to encourage her clients to call "every time they think they need something." A minister delivers a routine Sunday sermon, after which he makes himself unavailable to meet with several congregants troubled by the moral questions he raised for them. A therapist at a treatment center reprimands a child whose behavior has proven disruptive, focusing on consequences rather than understanding. In each of these instances, caregivers remove themselves from those needing their help. Careseekers are labeled and treated as parts, like the "gall-bladder" or the "troublemaker," rather than as more complex humans experiencing some difficult moment in their journeys toward growth and healing. They are dropped rather than held.

In short, people are more likely to fully receive care when they feel securely held by others. The notion of holding is central to effective caregiving relationships. British psychoanalyst D. W. Winnicott (1965) developed the concept of the holding environment to describe the nature of effective caregiving relationships between mothers and infants. Winnicott's insight was that "good-enough mothering" involves physically holding infants, whose subsequent experiences of feeling safely encompassed enable the initiation and movement of developmental processes. When mothers (or other primary caregivers) create reliably safe boundaries that protect infants from potentially disruptive stimuli, they enable their children to experience themselves as valued and secure (Winnicott 1960). They experience a protective space in which to safely examine and interact with what their worlds present, particularly when they are startled and temporarily need a secure base to which to retreat (Bowlby 1980). The reliable meeting of infants' physical needs – and later, of children's psychological needs – provides a way to develop and strengthen their egos and enable them to gradually learn to meet, in Winnicott's phrase, "the difficulties of life." Individual development is thus a gradual strengthening of one's capacity to handle environmental impingements. The child's ability to strengthen her ego is founded upon the original experience of being securely held (Balint 1968; Kohut 1977; Winnicott 1965).

The original holding environment is the mother's arms and all that enables those arms to be a safe place: the father's provision of an indestructible home and his enjoyment of the mother-child relationship, the lack of disruption from others, the physical space that presents comprehensible stimuli (Abram 1996; Winnicott 1960, 1965). The holding environment concept has been broadened to describe other settings, just as the secure base concept has been broadened to describe adult relations. The premise is the same: individuals, across their lives, will at times require places in which they can safely experience and work through difficulties. The concept was first broadened to describe the analytic setting, wherein therapists create environments in which patients are enabled to temporarily regress, to the point at which suppressed material is consciously processed (Balint 1968; Modell 1976; Winnicott 1965). The concept has more recently begun to be applied to a range of institutions, including residential treatment, healthcare, educational, and religious (Braxton 1995; Cohen 1984; Shapiro & Carr 1991). In these and similar caregiving organizations, holding environments allow careseekers to experience reliable caregiving.

Caregivers create holding environments through three types of behavior: containment, empathic acknowledgement, and enabling perspective (Kahn 2001). The three dimensions are drawn from clinical psychology (Kohut 1977; Rogers 1958; Winnicott 1960), group relations theory (Bion 1961; Shapiro & Carr 1991), organizational psychology (Kahn 1993), and philosophy (Noddings 1984).

Containment

Caregivers contain careseekers by making themselves accessible, actively inquiring about and attending to them, and receiving their experiences with compassion and acceptance. This allows caregivers to take in, to absorb, the experiences of those seeking their care, the better to understand their needs and how to meet them. When caregivers make themselves accessible to careseekers, they begin to contain parts of their experiences. A nurse sits momentarily with a patient, and takes in some of his pain. A teacher works with a group of struggling students, and takes in some of their confusion about a certain subject, and just beneath it, about their developing autonomy.

A social worker sits with a group of clients long enough to absorb some of their fear of and longing for control over their addictions.

What caregivers primarily absorb and contain are not thoughts but feelings. Careseekers, particularly those who experience anxiety, are not always able to put into words their own experiences. They are not able to say what kind of pain they are in, or how confused they are, or what their struggles are like. They communicate those experiences nevertheless, in word and tone and gesture. They do so by acting in ways, often enough, that will create in caregivers a state of mind similar to their own. It is a form of unconscious communication, known technically as projective identification (Klein 1959). An angry patient, unable to express that anger directly, will act in ways that infuriate the therapist, nurse, or physician. A sexually confused student will act in ways that send conflicting, confusing sexual messages to her teacher. A client who feels helpless and out of control in relation to his drug abuse habit will act in ways that leave his social worker feeling the same.

In such cases, careseekers unconsciously offload their states of mind onto others. They do so in the unarticulated wish to be rid of their anxiety. And they also wish for someone to contain, digest, reflect on, and offer back their experiences in ways that they too can digest and work with (Bion 1962; Klein 1959; Mawson 1994; Shapiro & Carr 1991). This dynamic is rooted in the infant's wish for the mother to hear his upset wailing, take in (and take away) his anger and confusion, understand his hunger or fear, and react in ways that will soothe and comfort. This wish to be contained carries through to adulthood. It is triggered by the experience of neediness. The confused students wish for someone to contain, reflect on, and speak to their confusion, just as the enraged abused youth in a residential center, the helpless addict, the disordered mental patient, and the fearful geriatric patient do. When caregivers are able to do so routinely, they are more likely to create the holding environments in which real work – the work of fully caring for others – may be accomplished. (When they cannot do so, they are subject to some of the stress detailed in Chapter 2.)

Empathic acknowledgement

Caregivers empathically acknowledge careseekers by curiously exploring their experiences, identifying with them, and validating them as they go about their attempts to grow, learn, or heal. To hold others well is to enable them to feel known, understood, and most important, valued. It is to enable them to feel cared for, not simply tended to as part of one's duties. When careseekers feel witnessed, in the deeper meaning of the word, they experience themselves as joined, as seen and felt, as known, and as not alone – the core experiences of feeling cared for (Noddings 1984). This is the layer of caregiving that exists below that of its more familiar components, namely, supporting others with appropriate resources, whether physical, emotional or technical (Mayeroff 1971; Memmi 1974). When careseekers are seen and validated, held by the attention and empathy of others, it is easier for them to receive care. They value themselves more. They forgive their own failures and half-steps more. They learn to witness and know themselves more deeply, and to care for themselves as they are cared for by others.

A childcare worker takes a long walk with a boy who has just instigated several fights with others in his residential dormitory. The worker is curious about what the fights were about, and the conversation moves gradually toward a discussion of the fights that routinely erupted in the boy's foster home. The worker does not judge the boy. He does not blame the boy. He inquires. The boy keeps talking. The childcare worker hears the boy's frustration and anger, and just beneath that, feels the boy's sadness. He tells the boy that he is doing remarkably well in not getting into more fights, given what he has been through. The boy nods, fighting back tears. They walk for some time in companionable silence. The worker tells the boy that he has the opportunity to do some wonderful things at the residential center; and that he, the worker, is very much looking forward to watching and helping and enjoying the boy's accomplishments. They keep talking as they walk back to the dormitory. They smile at one another as they part company.

This sort of interaction occurs in various forms in different caregiving institutions and relationships. Teachers sit with students and hear of their struggles and joys of mastering difficult academic material. Clergy lead discussions with congregants and learn of their searching questions and fears as they grow old or are faced with moral and spiritual issues for which they are not quite prepared. Therapists allow themselves to know, within their clinical hours, their patients, and validate the ways in which they have coped with, have ultimately survived, traumas of loss or abuse. Social workers travel to their clients' homes, sit with them, and learn, through the instrument of their own curiosity, how the clients have come to be in the places they are, and how they are not so very different from others whose fates have proven kinder. When caregivers are able to empathically identify with, and validate, the experiences of others, they help create holding environments.

Enabling perspective

Caregivers enable perspective for careseekers by helping them make sense of their experiences, orient toward what they need to do to achieve their goals, and interpret anxiety-arousing situations. Part of the caregiver's task is helping others get some distance from the anxiety and troubling emotions that threaten to overwhelm them. Containing careseekers and empathically acknowledging them provides support and sets the stage for them to take in their situations rationally. For them to actually do so, their own functioning egos will have to come into play. They will need to find ways to look past their anxiety and examine their situations and what might be done within them.

Caregivers help careseekers do this by joining with them to look at their situations and getting a useful perspective on them. This serves dual purposes: caregivers enable others to work through their current situations, and model for them the process of doing so.

This aspect of the holding environment, like the two others, appears in different forms in caregiving organizations but is inevitably a part of effective caregiving relationships. A nurse swings by the bed of a patient one afternoon with whom she had talked a fair amount in the days he had been in the unit. The patient had suffered a setback in his physical therapy a day earlier, having fallen twice during a session to strengthen his legs, which had suffered severe damage in an automobile accident. The nurse told the patient that she had heard about what happened. She asked him how he was feeling about it. The patient told her he was disappointed, and uncertain about whether he would ever return to normal. The nurse told him that what he was experiencing was in the normal course of events for an injury of his type. She now tells him that she understands how he might feel dejected – the man holds his head in his hands as she talks, barely looking up at her – and more, depressed. She then talks more about the physical therapy process, what happens with the muscles in the legs with his type of injury, and the likelihood of the process entailing more failures as he tries increasingly difficult movements. They talk together of how he might ask members of his family to his sessions, keep a journal of the process, or other ways he might prepare for these failures.

The seemingly simple, graceful ways in which the nurse helped her patient gain a perspective on his situation, as one climber helps another gain purchase on a difficult mountain slope by steadying him and focusing him on the task at hand, is found in other caregiving relationships as well. Teachers help students put into their proper place the nature and meaning of exams and papers. Social workers do the same for clients who are, say, newly involved in the criminal court system. Therapists and counselors do reality-testing with their clients, pointing them toward the facts rather than projections of troubling situations and what might be done to resolve them. Clergy members help congregants struggling with loss focus on the rituals, and what lies beneath them, to ease their pain. In such ways, direct caregivers steady those seeking their care, engaging their rational and thoughtful selves in the midst of the anxiety they carry.

Collectively, these three types of holding behavior enable careseekers to feel "safely overwhelmed" by events and situations. They enable people to let others take on their ego functioning while they themselves struggle with anxiety and difficult emotions (Klein 1987; Shapiro & Carr 1991). People allow themselves to simply be with (and at times be overwhelmed by) such emotions, knowing that they can temporarily lean on others. Caregivers provide an arms-around experience that allows for initiative and adventure

(Josselson 1992). They provide, in short, the secure base from which careseekers can venture forth toward their own growth, healing, and learning.

This lies at the heart of the work of caregiving organizations. Their primary tasks – teaching students, healing patients, ministering congregants, empowering the underserved, and the like – cannot be sustained in the absence of relationships of this type between direct caregivers and those who seek their help. It is the routine creation of secure, holding relationships that determines whether caregiving organizations are, in the deepest places of what they are and what they do, effective. It is this technology, that of the actual relationship of providing and receiving care as it appears in different guises in different institutions, that underlies the more observable techniques on display in those institutions. Finally, it is from this understanding of these kinds of organization that all else proceeds.

Implications for organizing

If the primary task of caregiving organizations best occurs through relationships between those who provide and those who receive care, then caregiving institutions must organize themselves to support these relationships. We thus need to examine how schools organize relationships between teachers and students, to ensure that the former create secure base relations with the latter, the better to support their efforts to master what they do not know. We would examine how residential treatment centers organize to ensure that clinical, residential and educational staff members integrate with one another and relate in a fully therapeutic manner with their clients. We would look to see how hospitals organize on behalf of the interactions between physicians and nurses and their patients; how churches and synagogues do so for relationships between clergy and congregants; and how others kinds of social service agencies and healthcare units do so for their own kinds of caregiving relationships.

In this formulation, caregiving relationships are at the center of the transactions between institutions and communities of careseekers. As part of their institutions, caregivers venture out toward careseekers, who are part of the larger communities in which the institutions exist. Together, they form temporary units with temporary boundaries, joining with one another for the purposes of providing and receiving some form of care, such as a lesson in mathematics, a medical procedure or treatment, a therapy session, a sermon or counseling session. They both remain connected to the larger groups they represent. The caregiver is the point of delivery of resources, support, and other aspects necessary to provide for the needs of careseekers. Behind them are the administrators, supervisors, and assorted departments and functions that, along with the group of direct caregivers, make up a caregiving institution. The careseeker is the point of reception.

For this process of delivering and receiving care to work effectively, caregiving organizations must find ways to take in their clients, symbolically if not literally, and work on their behalf. This process defines the nature of caregiving organizations, running beneath the observable work of teaching, ministering, nursing, guiding, and aiding. It is crucial to understand this process normatively if we are to analyze how and where these organizations fail in their intended work. Its three dimensions are described below.

Absorption

The needs of caregivers must be understood if they are to be fully served. If students, patients, clients, and the like are to be attended to based on what needs they actually present, the caregiving organization must organize to bring them in, in some fashion, and learn from and about them. The alternative is that members of caregiving organizations act on the basis of what they think they already know about those they serve: what they need, how they think and feel, how they will respond, what they will take in and what they will resist. The danger here is that of projection. Careseekers may be seen as caregiving organization members wish to see them, for reasons of their own, while the careseekers' actual needs will fade from sight, covered over by the organization's own unarticulated needs to treat them in certain ways.

Understanding careseekers' needs requires that they be *absorbed* in some fashion. They cannot simply be determined through focus groups or surveys. Careseekers are not always able to ascertain their own needs. Students may know that they need to learn certain material and pass certain courses but not that they need help in managing their social anxiety. Patients may know that they need specific operations or medication but not that their fears might disable them from following courses of treatment. Residential home youths might know that they have to stay out of trouble with the law but not that their rage is routinely triggered by feeling let down by figures of authority. The range of such needs, many of which exist beneath the surface of awareness, are crucial to understand if the caregiving relationship is to be effective as the core technology for the work.

Absorbing the range of careseekers' needs and experiences occurs in the context of the caregiving relationship itself. It requires some boundary separating the caregiving organization from its host community. Educators must bring students into school buildings, just as physicians must bring patients into hospital units, the better to work with them undisturbed by outside influences. At that boundary, caregivers create holding relationships with careseekers and in the process contain them. They absorb their experiences, their states of mind, and their emotions. They absorb information of which they are aware: the attitudes of students toward their academic work, congregants toward their spiritual dilemmas, patients toward their pain, clients toward their struggles to grow. They also absorb information of which they are unaware: careseekers' unconscious wishes, fears, and anxieties. A group of children and their parents struggling with bilingual education communicate their frustration and resentment by acting in ways that frustrate teachers and administrators. This is information communicated at a level *below* awareness.

Once absorbed, information about careseekers is inevitably imported into the caregiving organization. There, it must be extracted or unpacked from caregivers. It is only through such a process that reflection upon and learning about careseekers occurs. A caregiving organization is effective only to the extent that it organizes itself to engage this process. This involves creating settings for caregivers to discuss, reflect upon, and sift through their experiences of working with careseekers. It involves members throughout the organization valuing those experiences. It involves, in fact, holding caregivers – teachers, therapists, nurses and physicians, social workers, clergy members, and the like – at the center of their organizations, valued for what they contain about the careseekers. When these conditions are not met, careseekers' experiences remain contained within the caregivers, with ill effects on them and the work they and their organizations intend to do. When they are met, this sets the stage for the next part of the process.

Digestion

Once careseekers' experiences are available for scrutiny they must be worked with. They must be *digested* by organization members so they understand what, exactly, the careseekers are presenting for resolution. This is a complicated process. It involves not just the careseekers but also their communities, whose issues are suddenly re-presented within the organization. Often enough, caregiving organizations are asked to resolve issues in the communities in which they function; they are asked to hold, as it were, issues that cause anxiety in the community itself. Like underwater currents, these issues constantly influence what appears and moves on the surface of the work with students, clients, patients, and other careseekers.

Consider the example of the residential institution for the physically handicapped and the chronically sick. Miller and Gwynne (1972) describe two approaches to residential care. The "warehousing ideology" seeks to prolong physical life through medical and nursing care; residents are supposed to be passive and dependent, accepting their treatments from staff with neither protest nor displays of individuality. The "horticulture ideology" seeks to develop the capacities of individuals with unsatisfied drives and unfilled potential; residents are supposed to be active and striving, participating fully in their own ongoing development. As the authors note, both of these models are flawed, given the reality of residents' lives. The first model denies their autonomy; the second denies their dependence. Each residential institution must struggle with pressures toward each of these models, rooted as they are in communities and societies. The warehousing ideology reflects the belief that the handicapped are abnormal; they should be kept alive but they are not too much like normal people. The horticulture ideology reflects the belief that there are no differences between the disabled and the able-bodied, and that all that the former require is rehabilitation. The residential institution imports these contradictory beliefs. Its members must take them in on behalf of the larger community and find ways to reconcile them on behalf of their clients.

Caregiving organizations often struggle, as the residential institution does, with differing notions of their primary tasks. The issue of standardized testing in schools, for example, reflects a struggle over the primary task of public education: to develop the creative, critical faculties of individuals or to ensure the standardized equality of students. Hospitals might see-saw between the primary task of patient care versus that of profits, and in the case of teaching hospitals, between educating physicians, conducting funded research, and patient care. A social service agency working with abused children may struggle between the overt task of enabling their growth and the covert task of protecting them from their families.

Such conflicts in the definition of the primary task may emerge, as with the residential institution, from differing wishes in the community. They may also emerge from differing ideas within the organization about what its primary task ought to be, given various markets and sources of funding, as in the teaching hospital. The conflicts might also emerge from members' struggles with the emotions absorbed from the careseekers. The social service agency wishing to protect its clients (and perhaps undermining relations with the children's families who might otherwise be allies in the healing process) may be driven partly by the children's anxiety and rage, soaked up by the social workers. The work of clarifying an organization's primary task – which must occur if careseekers' needs are to be met in truly satisfying ways – is made more complicated by such emotions.

Since much gets absorbed at the boundary of the caregiving organization, its members must have the capacity to learn from rather than be overwhelmed by what it imports from the community and its careseekers. Its digestive system needs to be fully functional. This happens when caregivers, administrators, support staff, supervisors, and members of various departments and functions routinely revisit their primary task and their abilities to perform it effectively. Members need to express and confront the differing pulls, external and internal, acting on them to move away from their primary tasks. They need to negotiate their interpretations of their primary task. Finally, they need to decide together how they ought to work with careseekers to meet their needs. As the caregivers move back to the boundary at which they meet careseekers, they must be secure in the shared idea of their primary task and the type of relationship that best serves it. They need to be part of an organized system of caregiving that has absorbed and digested the careseekers' experiences and can re-present them in useful ways.

Provision

After absorption and digestion is *provision*. When information about care-seekers – their needs, experiences, states of mind, and emotions – has been made available for review and reflected on, organized caregiving may reasonably occur. It occurs through providing relationships between caregivers and careseekers. The relationships are organized – that is, they belong to and are anchored within the caregiving organization and its conception of the primary task, its structures and systems, its resources. The caregivers are contained within a system that supports their efforts to deliver care, in the relationships – between nurses and patients, teachers and students, social workers and clients, and other such pairings – in which careseekers' needs are met. Without such a system, caregivers are left adrift, unable to find purchase on solid ground as they are drawn into the currents of the careseekers' emotions. Organized caregiving enables perspective for the caregivers, supporting their efforts to offer perspective for others.

Consider again the organized caregiving of residential institutions for incurables. As Miller and Gwynne (1972) note, the ideal model for a residential institution is driven by neither the warehouse nor the horticulture ideology. Instead, it derives from the primary task of enhancing the resident's quality of life within the institution – that is, "to provide a setting in which he can find his own best way of relating to the world about him and to himself." Ideally, staff members who work in residential institutions serving the severely disabled can absorb and digest their clients' experiences enough to find their way toward articulating such a primary task. This opens the way for the creation of an organized system of caregiving supporting that task. In this case the organized system has three main components (Miller & Gwynne 1972). One set of activities focuses on caring for the residents, doing for them what they cannot do for themselves. A second set of activities focuses on *providing* residents with opportunities to satisfy their needs as independent individuals. The third set of activities supports residents, as with therapy and counseling, as they struggle with the pain of their situations. This organized caregiving system fits the institution's primary task. It anchors and guides the actions of all its members, particularly those who care directly for the residents.

These particular systems support the primary task of the residential institution for its population of incurables. Other systems support the primary tasks of the other types of caregiving organizations considered in this book. A school might well have specific academic activities that focus on teaching standardized material while reserving other activities for wildly creative, individualized instruction. The social service agency working with abused children might create forums in which the children can learn to both safely engage with and disengage from family members. A residential treatment center for drug abusers uses treatment teams as a primary vehicle, bringing together staff from education, therapy and residential treatment to integrate information and experiences on behalf of the residents. Each of these organizational structures and activities represents a way to provide care that serves the institution's understanding of its task, based on its members' absorption and digestion of its client population.

Insistent questions

The absorption, digestion, and provision cycle defines the work of caregiving organizations. It flows beneath the observable activities of teaching, ministering, and healing; it flows as well beneath the operations of the businesses that keep caregiving organizations financially viable. When this underlying process is disrupted in some fashion, caregiving organizations are less able to take in and respond to what lies around them, in their communities, and what lies within them, in their careseekers and in their staff; they are less able to work with what has been presented to them. They become inappropriately rigid, closed off from either their external or internal environments. Ideally, caregiving organizations are open systems, an idea developed by von Bertalanffy (1950) and elaborated by Rice (1963). Organizations, as open systems, need to import, convert and export materials in order to survive. Caregiving organizations must do so in the context of careseekers' needs and all that entails.

This framing leads to a set of questions that each caregiving organization must resolve. The questions are insistent. They will constantly re-present themselves, often in the form of increasingly troubling issues that tug at members, until satisfactorily resolved. The questions are: *How do we define our primary task, given the various definitions advocated by different groups within the community and within the organization? How do we take in information about the careseekers, their needs and states of mind? How do we deal with the emotions absorbed from careseekers, and those triggered by our work with them? How do we organize to support relationships between our caregivers and careseekers?* And, finally: *How do we insure that we revisit these questions and revise our answers as a matter of course?*

When these questions are not satisfactorily resolved, caregiving organizations develop telling symptoms. These include ongoing conflicts between departments, units, hierarchical levels, and functions; chronic burnout and turnover; patterns of staff members acting in inappropriate, unprofessional, or irrational ways; rifts between caregivers and administrators; the unwillingness of members to authorize leaders, or of leaders to collaborate with members or one another; and a chronic inability to make timely decisions, resolve problems, or develop and implement strategy. Each of these can be understood, of course, in terms of their own specific situations. Yet when they are persistent – when they do not yield to initial efforts to deal with the presenting symptoms – they are pointing to something more. Often enough, they point to some underlying disturbance in the organization's basic process of absorbing, digesting, and providing effectively for careseekers and their needs. They point to the unsatisfactory or non-existent resolution of the basic questions posed by the nature of the caregiving organization.

Caregiving organizations, like individuals beset by stress, often get disturbed and develop symptoms, as a matter of course. They are often in the difficult position of resolving issues – on behalf of individual careseekers and communities – for which there are no simple resolutions. Even when satisfactory resolutions are reached, they are not likely to remain effective over a long period of time. People's needs change as communities shift and the experiences and characteristics of students, clients, patients, congregants, and other careseekers evolve. The question of whether caregiving organizations will evolve as well, or whether they will remain stuck in patterns that are no longer useful to the true purposes of their work, is one, really, about resilience.

There will always be periods in which the patterns of thought and action in caregiving organizations lag behind the changes in careseekers and what they need. It is in those periods that the symptoms of underlying disturbances appear. This is a normal process in the ebbs and flows of caregiving organizations. It is what their members and leaders do during those periods that determine whether the disturbances remain. Resilient caregiving organizations are those in which such disturbances, and the symptoms pointing toward them, are diagnosed for what they are and treated as such.

Chapter 2

The stress of caregiving work

Stress is an inevitable byproduct of the caregiving task. Caring for others, in its various manifestations, places various forms of emotional, physical, and mental strain on people. It is exhausting to be constantly present for others, taking them in and helping them with their often difficult tasks of healing, growing, and learning. Parents know this instinctively. Raising children strains one's capacities. Lessons must be taught, values instilled, and emotions steadied during the ongoing transitions that mark a child's journey to young adulthood. Stress attends the daily ministrations – of food, advice, discipline, choices, and support – that characterize the parenting role. It occurs in key moments of transition or crisis, during which parents must struggle toward the right thing while managing their relationships with and reactions to their children. The caregiver's task is, in many ways, not so different from parenting. Caregivers are constantly working with people who regress in the service of receiving support or knowledge, of trying new ways of thinking and acting. They are engaged on a daily basis with dependent others. They must act within situations that contain transition or crisis with the possibility of great harm to others.

Caregivers are, of course, not careseekers' parents. They are hired to perform *jobs* – to teach, operate on, provide therapy to, counsel, conduct rituals for, or nurse others. They are not obligated to love others unconditionally; indeed, that would undermine their ability to perform their jobs effectively. They are obligated, however, to create relationships with careseekers in which the work of caregiving might be effectively performed. As discussed in the previous chapter, those relationships are the primary vehicle by which caregiving work is performed. Effective teachers do not simply impart information, as books do; nor do effective nurses, therapists, and physicians simply perform a set of techniques on the physical, emotional, or mental components of their patients, as a mechanic works on a broken car. The caregiving work occurs through relationships, between human beings who try to join together for that purpose. It is in the context of these relationships that the stress of caregiving work needs to be understood.

In this chapter I describe the various sources of stress that buffet the caregiving organization. I begin with those that affect the relationship between caregivers and careseekers, and then move on to discuss those that derive from the organizational and institutional contexts in which those relationships exist. The first order of stress is that felt by caregivers, who initially absorb much of the impact of working with clients, patients, students, and the like. The second order of stress is that experienced, in various forms, by all members of caregiving organizations. Each type of stress is related to its own factors, or stressors. A thorough understanding of these is crucial to an analysis of resilient caregiving organizations, for it is in the face of such stress that resilience occurs or gives way.

The strain of technique

The stressors that buffet caregiving organizations arrive at different depths. At the surface, like the waves of the ocean, is the stress associated with the techniques of caregiving. Different caregiving work depends on certain techniques. Therapists use specific techniques to elicit patients' experiences and emotions and enable insight. Nurses and physicians use various medical techniques to treat patients, dispense medication, and manage crises. Teachers develop and impart curricula through lectures, projects and exercises. Clergy use sermons, individual counseling, working with community groups on projects, and rituals. Social workers use counseling, interviewing, and legal skills to protect and support their clients.

Such techniques of caregiving require a certain level of skill and sophistication. They can often be quite demanding. A surgeon operating on a difficult case stands on his feet for over six hours, intensely concentrating, the scalpel in his hands moving precisely within an incision measured in fractions. A teacher struggles to create and deliver a lesson plan that teaches students about a difficult period in the history of her country, the impact of which continues to reverberate in the lives of the students and their families. A social worker confronts an alcoholic mother who stands in the door, refusing to let her child be examined in accordance with the latest court ruling. A minister counsels a couple whose marriage is slowly disintegrating over the undiscussed grief of a lost child. A therapist works with a group whose members slowly spin out of control, led by a vocal patient who has refused to continue taking his antidepressant medication. A childcare worker has to physically restrain a distraught, violent teenager whose parent has again missed a scheduled visit. A nurse darts from patient to patient on a busy medical ward, quickly checking their vital signs, updating their charts, and calling for assistance from attending physicians.

These tasks are not easy. They often require relatively high levels of physical, emotional, or mental stamina. That is stressful in its own right, particularly in situations where caregivers must perform with little respite: wards are crowded, surgeries or classes are scheduled one after another, caseloads are high, there are too many people to teach or heal and too many problems to take care of. During such periods – which in some organizations are relatively episodic, in others chronic – the workload itself adds its own layer of stress. One feels the press of time. There is too much to do and too little time in which to do it. There is little space for recovering one's balance before moving to yet another situation. The pace or the pressure of what needs to be done becomes a source of stress, separate from that associated with how one actually does the work.

There is also the stress associated with the potential for misapplied techniques. The costs of caregiving work done badly are quite high. Medical errors, with medications or surgical procedures, threaten lives. Social workers who cannot work effectively with violent families risk leaving children in abusive situations. Childcare workers know that those they work with might be teetering between lives of crime and lives of productive work, and that what sends struggling adolescents one way versus the other is often an attachment with an appropriately caring adult. Teachers can help instill or, alternatively, destroy their students' love of learning and intellectual engagement. Ministers, priests and rabbis can not only inspire congregants but also, through their lack of leadership or misconduct of their personal lives, turn congregants away from creating a rich religious life. Such caregivers understand the implications of their work, both that done well and that done poorly. They live and work with the constant knowledge that the techniques through which they serve others, performed unsafely or badly, can harm others irreparably. This knowledge presses down upon them. They are most aware of its press, of course, when they find themselves in situations that threaten danger to careseekers. But it is constant, always just behind their consciousness. It is part of their world, like the air they breathe, and it exerts its strain.

The strain of absorption

Those who work directly with clients, patients, students, and congregants are also subject to the stress of absorbing them. As discussed earlier, people's needs, experiences, and emotions must be taken in and understood if they are to be cared for in effective, lasting ways. They must be absorbed by caregivers, who represent them (or, more literally, "re-present" them, voicing their presence) in the organization. Such representation occurs only to the extent that caregivers take in careseekers. This taking in of others – of fully grasping what they know and how they know it, what they fear and are excited about, what their needs and wishes really are – occurs through the creation of relationships. These are often a source of stress, in two primary ways. First, the stress derives from what is actually absorbed by caregivers in their work with others. Second, it derives from the process of creating and maintaining the relationships through which that absorption occurs.

What caregivers absorb depends on what careseekers carry with them into their interactions. This varies with the task of the organization, and what that task evokes in people served by that organization. In schools the task is to educate students, introducing them to a body of widely accepted knowledge and imparting the skills by which to access, learn, and add to that knowledge. This task raises student anxiety related to the fear of not being able to learn, of being left behind, of being unable to join the rest of the society as a fully-fledged member. It also evokes anxiety, confusion, shame, wonder, and the ambivalence of wanting both social acceptance and individual self-assertion. In hospitals, mental health facilities and wards, clinics and treatment centers, the task is to heal patients, which evokes anxiety about survival and death, physical and mental incapacitation. They are anxious about the process of treatment, the pain it might entail, and its outcomes, the various types of scars that might be left upon or within them. In social service agencies serving under-served populations that have few resources or ways of garnering support, the clients are frightened and anxious about what will happen to them and, often enough, traumatized by what has already happened. They may feel displaced and unwanted, in pain, isolated and angry, afraid; beneath that, they may be ashamed and guilty. In residential treatment organizations, residents are often enraged, while longing to be cared for. They may be sad, perhaps depressed, and ashamed or guilty, as if their actions caused them to be taken away from their communities. They may be confused about how they ended up in these circumstances, and about how to find their way to some other, better place in their lives. They are often distrustful of those around them.

In nursing homes, geriatric inpatient wards, and senior citizen centers, the emotional undercurrents are marked by a pressing awareness of death. This awareness, conscious and not, evokes particular responses in the aged. It evokes fear, of course. It also evokes anticipation (of release from pain and memory), guilt and remorse (over what was done and not done in one's life), anger (at one's infirmity), sadness (for the relationships with others and one's own self that are coming to an end), and longing (for more time for those relationships). For some, there is also a sense of peace and appreciation, and a period of reflection. Finally, in religious institutions – churches, temples, ministries, and other houses of worship – that minister to people's spiritual needs, congregants may be anxious about the larger issues related to existential meaning, the conduct of moral lives, and the place, meaning and outcome of death in one's life. They may be uncertain and confused about the definition of a good life, one that balances the pursuit of earthly matters with conduct that is moral and principled. And there are also the emotions that attend people's apprehension and experiences of God in their lives: longing, confusion, frustration, awe, disbelief.

Each of these careseeker populations carries with it some form of distress, whether it be anxiety, confusion, sadness, or some other disturbing emotion.

Caregivers routinely work with distressed people seeking relief. Such distress creates an encompassing layer of stress with which caregivers must cope. The stress itself derives from the constant waves of emotions that wash up against caregivers as they perform the technical tasks of their work with careseekers. It is draining to work with upset and anxious students, frightened patients, distressed addicts, furious adolescents, bitter seniors, or others who are in great distress. To get close enough to learn about careseekers and what they need, caregivers come squarely up against careseekers' emotions. Absorbing useful knowledge about careseekers is not simply a transmission of information; transmitted also is the careseekers' experiences and feelings about those experiences. Skilled caregivers learn, of course, to develop filters. They learn to develop boundaries permeable enough to establish a necessary relationship with distressed others, yet impermeable enough to hold onto the quite real distinctions between themselves and others. This allows caregivers a form of *detached concern*: they identify with those seeking their care, but not so much that they lose sight of their role. They bring others in emotionally but limit the depths of that entry such that they remain their own, separate people, filled with the purposes of their roles rather than with the experiences of those they need to serve.

Yet even with the skill of detached concern, working with distressed people is stressful. When teachers, therapists, social workers, healthcare workers and ministers take in others emotionally in the context of their work, they inevitably absorb others' emotions and experiences. They take in others' sadness, fear, anger, and anxiety. Some remain filled in such ways, particularly those who have not yet learned to limit the depth of their relations with students, clients and patients; they learn, slowly, to extricate themselves from others, emotionally. If they do not, they develop compassion fatigue (Figley 1995), becoming so filled with others' emotions that they cannot absorb any more. Others clear themselves more quickly, through ongoing supervision, peer networks, and forms of self-expression and self-care. Either way, the process takes its toll. It is difficult to remain a caregiver and not get worn by the effort to clear oneself emotionally. As containers become worn with repeated use, so do caregivers tire of the process of connecting to and then moving away from careseekers. As containers build up residue of what they have contained, many times over, so do caregivers contain within them a lasting memory and experience of others' distress. The proximity to pain and distress takes its toll.

The strain of relationship, Part I

The stress of absorption derives not simply from what careseekers contain, in the form of distress and difficult emotions, but from the relational process itself. Relationships with careseekers may be quite difficult, for perfectly understandable reasons. They often require a great deal of time. Therapists must sit with patients long enough, and patiently enough, to earn their trust;

their attention must be unwavering enough to enable patients to feel valued or understood. Teachers must do the same, fashioning connections with each of their students in order to enable them to feel individually attended to. Nurses and physicians need to connect with their patients, enough to learn what they need, where they hurt, the history of their symptoms, what they understand of their illnesses. Such relational work often occurs in contexts not always perfectly conducive to the investment of time necessary: caregivers may be required to care for too many people in not enough time, with not enough resources.

The underlying source of the difficulty of creating ongoing relationships with careseekers is related less to logistics, however, than to *anxiety*. Put sharply, when people are in distress, acute and chronic, it is not an entirely simple or, for that matter, pleasurable matter to be in close relationship with them. They may be too anxious to settle easily into the caregiving relationship. They may act out that anxiety in ways that may make it difficult for them to get their needs met. The patient with a life-threatening disease, terrified, withdraws from her treatment, missing appointments and medication. The recovering addict, anxious about his ability to survive, tries to emotionally blackmail his social worker, threatening to go back to his drugs unless she meets certain demands. The student with enormous family pressure for academic success pushes her teachers to give her better grades. The congregant whose spouse is battling depression attaches herself to the minister, begging him to simply tell her what to do to fix the problem. The child who has been removed from an abusive home, afraid to get close to others who might also hurt or abandon him, remains defiant and unyielding in his relations with childcare workers.

Careseekers thus present their responses to their situations, sometimes directly through their words, but mostly in how they act in relation to caregivers. They act skittish, upset, or afraid; they are arrogant and condescending, trying to control and mask their fear but holding others at some remove; they cling, attaching themselves as if drowning to others as if they were life-preservers. Any or all of such actions confront caregivers. They are both expressive (people expressing their experiences) and defensive (people attempting to move away from conscious experiences of pain, anxiety, and distress).

It is the defensive function that puts particular strain on caregivers, as people try to rid themselves of their distress by acting in certain ways in relation to their caregivers. They may divide the contradictory feelings into differentiated, often polarized elements (splitting), and then locate one side of polarity onto others (projection) (Freud 1936; Klein 1959; Smith & Berg 1987), as when a patient undergoing chemotherapy projects onto the nurse the sense of hopefulness, often telling her how "upbeat" she is, while he focuses on morbidity statistics, his seemingly worsening condition, and a sense of pervasive dread. They may regress, attempting to return to earlier libidinal stages of functioning in order to avoid psychological tension or conflict that gets evoked at present levels of functioning (Kaplan & Sadock 1989), as when a student facing a difficult set of final exams avoids studying completely, insists that the exams did not matter and blames the teacher for the unfairness of the exams. They may become passive-aggressive, in which aggression toward others is expressed indirectly through passivity, maso-chism, and turning against one's self (Kaplan & Sadock 1989), as when a cancer patient, furious at his wife for leaving him, stops taking medication and keeping appointments. Or they may "act out," expressing their unconscious impulses and wishes through actions that let them avoid being conscious of painful affect (Kaplan & Sadock 1989), as when a child in the residential treatment center whose mother missed yet another visiting appointment flings his tray of food at the cafeteria wall, is physically restrained by two childcare workers, and feels, in the ensuing struggle, physically held and not alone.

When careseekers employ such defense mechanisms, they exact a toll on caregivers. The caregivers may be the objects on which projections are made: they are treated as if they were brutal, unconditionally loving, rigid, untrustworthy, or other one-dimensional labels that restrict their abilities to work effectively. Caregivers may be the ones with whom careseekers regress. They must then figure out how to appropriately support careseekers, to minister to their distress, without being drawn into others' regressive dramas. Caregivers may also have to deal with others refusing, in their passive-aggressiveness, to care for themselves. Or they may have to deal with others acting out, harming themselves or others in order to avoid painful affect. There is a significant level of stress here for caregivers who come into contact with people who routinely employ such defense mechanisms. They must sim-ultaneously protect themselves from being harmed by those defenses while creating the relationships in which others can effectively heal, learn, grow, and change. They must absorb assaults.

It is not always like this, of course. Many careseekers do not routinely employ defense mechanisms. They simply go about the business of being students, patients, clients, congregants, and the like, doing their best to accomplish their goals and move on. They try to create reasonably healthy relationships with their teachers, therapists, social workers, healthcare work-ers, and ministers. They are often successful in doing so. Yet, even so, there is strain attached to these relationships that affects caregivers. The strain comes from the seemingly inevitable action of *transference* that attends caregiving relationships. The classic definition of transference derives from psycho-analysis. Sigmund Freud conceptualized it as the patient's experience of feel-ings toward the analyst that do not befit the analyst *per se* but belong to an earlier person from the past, someone who was a central figure in the patient's affect-laden early years of life (Freud 1977). Typically, this was a parent, or some other central caregiver. Transference is thus an intrapsychic process that becomes an interpersonal one: the patient acts toward the therapist as if that therapist was the patient's father, mother, or other major figure in his or her internal life.

Transference occurs quite normally in caregiving relationships. It is not limited to the psychoanalytic or psychotherapeutic setting. It is often triggered by people's reactions to those in authority. It is quite common for people to have transferential reactions to their teachers, therapists, physicians, clergy, nurses or social workers. As caregivers they symbolically represent earlier figures in people's lives. People instinctively map parent-child relationships onto caregiving relationships. It is our first model of relationship. When we enter situations in which we require some form of support or assistance – the classroom, sanctuary, hospital, therapist's or physician's office, social service agency – we are predisposed to map onto those situations the internal terrain we know so intimately: our parent-child relationships. We look to our caregivers as we once used to look toward our parents. It is our instinct. In acute pain, we cry out for our mothers, our fathers, those who loved and held us, well or poorly, when we were very young. In the normal distress of the careseeker we are predisposed to see caregivers through the same lenses as we saw our earliest caregivers.

Caregivers thus often experience others acting as children in relation to them as parents. People of all ages seem to regress when they assume the roles of students, patients, congregants, and clients. This is a double-edged sword. On the one hand, such regression is necessary for people to allow others to teach, minister to, and in other ways work with them. On the other hand, such regression may present itself as abject dependence, in which careseekers are overly submissive, helping to create relationships that emphasize the caregivers' knowledge and expertise and diminish their own. Or the regression may present as counter-dependence. People may deny their needs for assistance from or resist the authority of teachers, healthcare workers, ministers and others caregivers. When careseekers draw on the parent-child model, as they inevitably do, they thus regress in ways that may or may not be useful to what they seek to accomplish. They may work with or against the creation of useful, secure relationships with caregivers.

The strain of creating relationships with careseekers is related, in many ways, to the fact that caregivers happen to populate environments that are particularly evocative for careseekers. The needs of careseekers evoke in them emotions of one sort or another: longing, fear, joy, sadness, anxiety. The settings in which they seek to meet those needs evoke the unconscious, internal models they have of their earliest caregiving relationships. The therapist and the teacher, social worker and nurse, physician and minister: they are the screens upon which others' emotions, needs, wishes, and longings are projected, without awareness. Caregivers must wade through these almost impossibly deep waters daily, simply to get close enough to others to do their jobs. This is stressful work as it involves the daily construction of relationships with people often distracted by external circumstances and their own internal worlds.

The strain of relationship, Part II

Relationships are fed by tributaries of emotions, needs, wishes, and capabilities streaming in from all parties. In caregiving organizations, relationships between careseekers and caregivers are shaped not simply by the characteristics and responses of the former. Caregivers themselves contribute a fair amount to the interactions as well. They are not simply machinists who stand in one place as the assembly line flows past, stamping raw material with barely a passing glance or thought. Caregivers use their thoughts and their feelings to guide them in their work with others who need their help. Therein lies both the promise and the difficulty of their work. The promise is that of using the self – one's own reactions, thoughts, and feelings – as a source of information, a receiver of sorts, through which one absorbs and digests a great deal about those one seeks to help. The difficulty is related to the fact that, as receivers, we are imperfect. We routinely register information that may derive from within our own selves, not others. We react to information that seeps up from somewhere within us, rather than (or in combination with) information we pick up in our sensing of others. We are not often aware of doing so.

Ideally, caregivers use their selves to receive others' transmissions as a matter of course. People in distress are not always able to directly verbalize their experiences. Children may not be able to tell teachers that they are feeling an inordinate amount of pressure at home, tell social workers they are afraid to go home to their foster parents, or tell their therapists of their rage or sadness at being abused or left by their parents. Adult patients are not always able to express their anxiety about their treatments, what they will entail or whether they will work. Recovering addicts may not be able to articulate the guilt they feel about all those they have left, and let down, in their lives. This is important information for caregivers to have; it enables them to understand what others contain within them that may facilitate or undermine efforts to receive help and engage in their own growth and healing. Yet although careseekers are not always able to verbalize their experiences, they do communicate them, as noted in the previous chapter, through the unconscious process of projective identification (Bion 1962; Hinshelwood 2001; Segal 1981).

When individuals act in ways that deposit aspects of themselves in others, they exert pressure on others to experience feelings similar to those that they contain within themselves (Obholzer & Roberts 1994; Shapiro & Carr 1991). The child who feels upset by being pressured at home pressures the teacher, enabling her to feel similarly upset. The fearful adolescent intimates violence in his relations with his social worker, who becomes afraid in precisely the way that the adolescent does at home. The enraged or depressed youth acts in ways that lead his therapist or childcare worker to feel angry at or sad with him. The anxious surgical patient badgers the nurses and physicians, making them anxious as well. The addict tries to make her social worker feel guilty for her plight, as she herself feels guilty about those she has betrayed. These are each communications, of a sort. They occur wordlessly, at the level below direct expression. They use a primitive language that predates verbalization: it is the language of the wailing infant who cries in order to communicate to his mother his distress. Ideally, as Winnincott (1960) noted, the mother absorbs the infant's cries, feels distress, and moves to care for the child until the distress dissolves. Such is the unexpressed, unconscious wish of careseekers: that caregivers will absorb that which pains them, interpret and understand the messages transmitted within the distress, and act to relieve distress.

Caregivers thus need to unpack through self-reflection what has been deposited within them by others' projective identifications. They must unpack their emotions and experiences as one might unpack a suitcase, carefully laying out and examining its contents. They must reflect on what they feel as a matter of course; they must dispassionately examine their reactions to certain people and events. This is a technical matter, related to caregivers' abilities to practice the discipline of self-reflection. Others' projections and defenses are not simply to be rejected, dismissed, or defended against. They are to be made sense of. They are to be understood as messages from the parts of people that cannot come forth in verbal expression. This requires that others be absorbed well enough that they emotionally "get to" their caregivers – but not so much that caregivers are disabled by being "gotten to" so much.

This work is stressful partly because of the imperfection – or rather, the humanity – of the caregivers themselves. Caregivers are not immune to having their own experiences of the situations of others, independent of what is projected upon them. What gets evoked within careseekers – dread and anxiety in relation to sickness and death, for example, or helplessness and anger in relation to social inequity – is often evoked within the caregivers themselves. Nurses, physicians, and other healthcare workers may react to others' fear of pain, incapacitation, and death with their own anxiety, their own pity, compassion, and guilt. Social workers may feel guilty in relation to their clients. Clergy may feel anxious about their own doubts as they minister to others seeking answers to often unanswerable questions. Teachers may have their own unresolved anxiety about competence and social acceptance. This is stressful for caregivers, as both others' and their own anxieties lay siege. It is particularly stressful when what gets stirred up within caregivers is related to the parts of themselves that identify with careseekers, or put another way, to the parts of themselves that *are* careseekers.

Understanding this formulation depends on a sophisticated realization of the motivations of many of those who devote their lives to helping others grow, heal, and learn. People are often drawn to the caring professions because of a need for reparation: "to put something right," in Dartington's (1994) phrase, in relation to what had been not right in their own early experiences. People are drawn to certain professions, clients, and settings by their need to come to terms with unresolved issues from the past (Roberts 1994a). The wish is that the job situation will resolve early life situations that feel unsettled, that were and continue to be a source of emotional wounds. The child for whom there was little maternal care learned to care for herself, and for those around her, and continues to do so as a nurse, therapist, physician, or social worker. The child who grew up in a family that could not, finally, hold together becomes a therapist or social worker, intervening with other families. The child subjected to abuse finds himself drawn to residential care settings to work with others who have been abused. The child who felt incompetent or slow, or who longed for others to teach her while teaching herself, becomes a teacher of others.

Such people may be drawn to the scene of the crime, as it were. They return to settings in which they were profoundly dissatisfied or distressed in the unconscious hope that they can have a different experience. They unconsciously wish to repair and make right that which was not right. They hope to have unmet needs finally met. They wish to protect others from having experiences similar to their own. Or, finally, they wish to undo what had been done to them, which can only occur, seemingly, by ministering to others. Their own development was halted at some place or another, and they return to settings in which they can be part of a continued development, even if it is not their own. There are also those, of course, who are drawn to the caring professions for precisely the opposite reason: they were cared for well, and they wish to similarly care for others. For these people, caregiving work is an expression of gratitude for good care received. Often, however, caregivers consciously believe that they fall into this latter category while in fact they are driven by their unconscious desires for reparation. This is also true, though perhaps less powerfully, for administrators and staff who, while not working directly as caregivers, may find themselves drawn, as if responding to a gravitational pull, toward settings in which they are able to experience, if only vicariously, "good-enough" caring relationships.

Such unconscious motivations heighten the possibility for *counter-transference* on the part of caregivers. Counter-transference occurs when the unconscious needs, wishes, and conflicts of caregivers are evoked by those with whom they work and brought into interactions in ways that influence, often negatively, objective judgment and reason (Kaplan & Sadock 1989). The teacher finds herself enraged with a few of her male students for acting unruly, which unconsciously evokes her anger at being the "teacher's pet" for much of her own life as a student. The therapist is attracted to his vivacious patient, who evokes in him a suppressed longing for authentic expression in his life. The nurse feels overwhelming sadness and guilt over a dying patient, feelings that originated much earlier in her life in relation to a father who died when she was young. Such emotional reactions seem to be about the care-seekers, or about the settings, but they are, finally, about what is contained within the caregivers themselves. The caregivers place themselves in certain settings in order to be able to release those feelings. They need to do so: feelings demand expression, and if they cannot be expressed directly and in relation to the events and settings from which they originated, then they will be in relation to events and settings substituted for that purpose.

This process has several significant implications for caregiving work and workers. First, counter-transference makes it difficult to decipher the primitive language by which careseekers communicate their experiences to others. A childcare worker's sudden anger or deepening sadness is related to his own unresolved experiences, but has been triggered by some event or situation with a child. It might not have much to do with the child's experiences or what he may be trying to communicate. Ghosts are disturbed within the childcare worker. They will haunt her until they have had their say and been laid to rest. Meanwhile, they are noisy, sending up a din within the childcare worker that makes it difficult for her to hear the child's communications.

Second, caregivers undermine their work when they over-identify with careseekers. They may engage in their own projective identifications, projecting onto others the suppressed parts of themselves that cannot find direct expression – the abused, wounded, angry, depressed, fearful, anxious, curious, or risk-taking parts of themselves. They may then relate to others in terms of what they wish to see about them. They relate to the projected part of themselves, rather than to others as separate individuals. This gets in the way of absorbing others on their own terms. They cannot easily reinforce careseekers for expressing the parts of their selves that do not conform to the projective identifications. If nurses wish to see their patients as helpless, the better to believe that they are themselves completely in control, it is difficult for them to encourage their patients' autonomy. If teachers wish to see their students as knowing less, the better to believe they are themselves smart and knowledgeable, it is difficult for them to reinforce their students' burgeoning intellects. They operate, in Jungian terms, from the shadows of their projections, from which they may be unconsciously destructive to others (Guggenbuhl-Craig 1971).

Finally, caregivers may set for themselves "impossible tasks" (Roberts 1994a) rooted more in their internal needs than in the missions of their organizations. A childcare worker at a residential treatment center tries to ensure that his young clients are protected from any interaction with their parents. A nurse at a geriatric facility wants patients to experience absolutely no pain. A social worker working with a state agency tries to make sure that all families remain intact, regardless of particular circumstances. Such efforts are fruitless, in the practical sense. They are also inordinately stressful, since they cannot be accomplished. They are often inappropriate to the primary tasks of the caregiving organizations themselves. These caregivers have substituted different tasks, emanating from their own unconscious needs and wishes for reparation. Such reparation is, often enough, manic rather than genuine. Manic reparation is driven by the unconscious wish for total redemption; as Roberts (1994a: 116) writes, workers "unconsciously hope to confirm that they have sufficient internal goodness to repair damage in others," so as not to experience the anxiety, guilt, grief, or other emotions lodged within them from earlier experiences. Genuine reparation, on the other hand, "requires the ability to face that damage has been done and cannot be undone" (Roberts 1994a: 116). Here, caregivers are able to accept what they can and cannot reasonably do, for they have accepted what was and was not done for them. If they cannot do so, they will wage an ongoing, stressful and ultimately unsuccessful campaign to repair that which cannot be repaired.

The strain of creating and maintaining caregiving relationships is thus related not simply to how distracted careseekers are by their circumstances but by how distracted caregivers themselves are as well. Caregivers need to maintain a certain hard-won clarity about their own side of the relationship, even as they assume some responsibility for absorbing and getting clear about the other side. They need to observe their selves, and clear their selves emotionally, the better to make room for taking in and understanding others. They need to do this while being buffeted by strong emotional undercurrents – their own, careseekers' – that flow toward one another and create number-less waves, cross-currents, depths, and pulls toward and away from useful, caring encounters.

Contextual strains

Caregiving organizations, and the societies in which they function, are the cause of some strain as well, not simply for caregivers but for other organiza-tion members as well. One source of stress is increasingly the lack of resources that characterize many caregiving organizations. Caregiving organ-izations are often struggling for resources, financial and human, and in losing those struggles, members are asked to do a lot with too little. Caregiving organizations must, like corporations, struggle to contain costs, deliver profits or high margins, raise funds, increase market share, and operate with an eye on remaining solvent. Hospitals, schools, churches, social service agencies and the like are increasingly involved in the fundraising business. They are also in the business of creating financially sound organizations in which budgets and all that they entail – justifications for spending, containing costs, reducing overheads, cutting services and programs – are increasingly central and important.

The stress here hits different members in different ways. Administrators experience the strain of having to operate in a context of scarce resources. Their roles require them to think and act strategically, to navigate their enterprises through uncertain, often inhospitable markets. School super-intendents and principals must develop ways to allot monies that cover some but not all basic services, and raise other monies from their communities. Directors of social service or welfare agencies that serve the public must consistently develop strategies based on their readings of the shifts of political winds. Hospital administrators must develop strategies that attract patients, physicians, and researchers in quite competitive markets. The strain of this work is located not simply in the tasks themselves. It also derives from the anxiety attached to maintaining the ongoing survival of organizations that, unlike many corporations, have little access to ready sources of funding.

Caregivers, for their part, experience the strain of scarce resources in terms of increasing demands. Teachers face more crowded classrooms. Social workers and therapists have larger caseloads. Healthcare workers see more patients in less time in order to meet productivity requirements. Clergy have less staff to help with the duties of their offices. These caregivers are forced to create swifter relationships with careseekers. They feel tugs away from spend-ing the time with others that allows them to take them in more fully, to absorb and digest them as they need to be digested. It is, often enough, only through conscious acts of will that they resist these tugs. When they cannot, caregivers experience both the conscious stress of their caseloads, and the deeper, more insidious stress of their failure to serve all those who come to them for help in their efforts to grow, learn, and heal. The stress is often not mitigated by caregivers developing realistic rather than overly ambitious goals in relation to careseekers (Lyth 1988).

The strain of scarce resources is joined by the stress of change, as leaders search this way and that to fit the pieces of the puzzle – markets, services, personnel, costs – into a strategic, viable picture. The medical unit director decides to merge her unit with another. The school head decides to create a new curriculum to attract new funding. The senior administrators of a resi-dential treatment center move to close down the girls' house and concentrate only on adolescent boys. The minister begins to rally congregants to begin a ministry for the homeless. Such change churns anxiety. Organization members are uncertain about what the changes will mean for them; they do not know how their jobs or lives will change. The uncertainty is exacerbated for people who feel left out of the change process. Direct caregivers, often busy providing services, are often relatively isolated from other members, particularly administrative leaders, and experience that isolation as power-lessness. That sense is heightened when caregivers lack the authority within their organizations to make policy changes they believe will best serve careseekers.

There is a larger context here as well. Caregiving organizations contain the uncertain, often contradictory demands of the societies in which they operate, and caregivers must wade daily through such contradictions. Teachers are asked to develop individual students' potentials while using curricula and standardized tests that press toward homogenization. Counselors working with drug and alcohol abusers must find and lose and find again the proper balances of punishing and supporting their clients. Nurses working in geriatric health units must deal with the tensions between their desires to rehabilitate and the families' desires to warehouse their patients. Physicians must deal with the terrible choices about who to enroll in experimental drug protocols, balancing the pulls toward helping all patients with the need for scientific experimentation requiring placebo groups. Such tensions originate in society but become firmly located within the organizations themselves. They result in incompatible objectives and conflicting task definitions. They become located within and between organization members and their groups, which then wage battles on behalf of the societies that they serve. There is a fair amount of stress involved here. It rarely lessens, for societal contradictions remain unresolved and their mandates remain ambiguous. They become another backdrop, and a stressful one at that, for caregiving work.

Holding on, letting go

Members of caregiving organizations live and work with these strains daily. At times they rise sharply and threaten to overwhelm into crises. Mostly they are simply there, pressing down steadily. The pressure is greatest on direct caregivers. It is in their relationships with clients, patients, students, and congregants that many of the strains are located or evoked, yet pressure also exists for other members who work amidst steady streams of uncertainty, ambiguity, and anxiety related to the task and what it evokes in careseekers and their communities. The key question here is how members, particularly caregivers, react to the strain. Do they hold on to the caregiving tasks of their organizations (and thus to careseekers, and to one another), or do they let go and turn away, like exhausted swimmers who halt their seemingly futile attempts to swim against the current?

What distinguishes the two, primarily, is the question of how members collectively choose to respond to the strains that attend their work. More precisely, it is how they choose to work with the emotions that flow through their organizations. Beneath the observable, daily work of teaching, counseling, nursing, ministering, and the like lies the emotional life of an organization, running underground like a deeply-fed spring. Emotions flow in with the clients, and from the caregivers themselves. They create currents of a sort. How members respond to those currents – and in particular, whether they lash themselves together and ride them out, or let the currents split them apart – determines the resiliency of their organizations. Chapter 3 describes the nature of such resiliency.

Chapter 3

Resilience under stress

Some caregivers cannot maintain effective caregiving relationships. To alleviate the stress of the work, they tumble into inappropriately close relations with others in order to meet their own needs. Or they distance themselves too far from others in order to protect themselves. They burn out, becoming emotionally unavailable, listless, or hardened. Other caregivers are able to maintain the right balance – close enough to absorb, distant enough to maintain perspective and others' autonomy – and hold onto rather than let go of their primary task of helping others. They ride out the inevitable points of stress that threaten to destabilize them and their work. These caregivers are resilient. They are able to return to a steady state of balanced relationship – that paradoxical stance of simultaneous openness to and detachment from those they seek to help – after being temporarily laid low by the stress of their experiences of the other, the difficulty of their work, their own emotional reactions, a sense of hopelessness, or some other disturbance. They are flattened, momentarily out of commission, and then they regain their shape and return to their work and relationships.

Resilience is "the capacity to rebound from adversity more strengthened and more resourceful. It is an active process of endurance, self-righting, and growth in response to crisis and challenge" (Walsh 1998: 4). Individuals are tested in some form or another, they endure suffering, and they emerge stronger from the experience. They are not invulnerable or impervious to adversity. Rather, they "struggle well," in the words of Froma Walsh (1998), a family therapist who has written on resilience in the context of family systems. Such resilience may be understood in individual terms. Some people seem to have the ability to quickly bounce back from difficult, stressful situations. They assess a situation, do what they need to do to understand its dimensions and act effectively within it, let go of that over which they have little control, and move on. Through quirks of personality, or experience, or history they are simply more resilient than others. They have relatively high self-esteem, and a realistic sense of hope and personal efficacy. They are confident that odds can be surmounted, optimistic in their abilities to shape events.

Yet resilience is also very much a matter of context. Walsh (1998) has summarized a great deal of research indicating that resilience occurs within, and is shaped by, relational and systemic contexts. She cites studies indicating that people are more resilient when they have greater access to caring others. Children who had at least one person who accepted them unconditionally, to whom they could turn when they needed to, with whom they could identify, and from whom they could gather strength were able to overcome hardships (Werner 1993; Werner & Smith 1992). This relational principle may be further generalized. Families may be understood as a set of relations which create systems that are more or less resilient. Family resilience refers to coping and adaptational processes that mark the family as a functional unit. Families vary in their ability to mediate stress and enable members to surmount crises. As Walsh notes, "Ongoing family processes can boost immunity to stress, preventing or reducing harmful impact. Family processes can be rallied as resources to compensate for negative stress effects" (1998: 19). How a family confronts and manages stress thus shapes how its members, and itself as a unit, adapts to adverse situations.

The same may be said for caregiving organizations. As described in the previous chapter, caregivers and other organizational members are subjected to ongoing layers of stress that, cumulatively, create conditions of hardship and adversity. Members may suffer in the face of the ongoing tide of care-seekers' emotions and what they evoke. They may experience trauma through the accumulation of daily pressures and crises or the eruption of larger events – the accidental death of a child in a hospital ward, a stabbing in a school, allegations of abuse by a staff member – that have the potential to leave them reeling. They may be tempted to regress, burn out, disengage, or act out. What they actually experience, however, or what they actually do in relation to those experiences, has much to do with the resilience of their organizations. Like couples, families, and communities, caregiving organizations vary in their ability to prevent and cope with stress; they vary in their ability to create the conditions enabling their members to "struggle well" in the face of the daily stress of institutional life.

In the most resilient organizations, members deal cleanly with stress and trauma. A group of school administrators and teachers meet in the wake of an incident in which a teenager was caught with a knife in school. A medical unit develops a program for reporting and solving medical errors and near-misses. A social service agency examines the sudden rise in social workers' absenteeism and turnover. A residential treatment center struggles to under-stand the latest outbreak of clients' violence toward staff and staff responses. A government-funded clinic develops a strategy to cope with drops in funding. In such circumstances, members face squarely the source of their difficulties. They talk about them, act together to alter their circumstances, remain positive and hopeful about their abilities to influence their environ-ments. They mourn or grieve the losses they face. They grow stronger. They grow closer to one another in the context of their work together. They cope, they adapt, and they move on rather than remain paralyzed and ineffective. They are resilient.

Resilient caregiving organizations are marked by members joining with one another to create *caregiving systems*, each of which is a series of integrated units whose members work together across boundaries to respond to the needs of careseekers. Primary caregivers are the vehicles through which care is actually delivered, but the care itself is drawn from the joint workings of members across their organizations. Caregivers are the most visible parts of a caregiving system but are not the system itself. They are the points of delivery. What they deliver – knowledge, expertise, support, caring – exists in the organization itself, like pools from which caregivers draw to replenish themselves as they engage those who seek their care.

Thus, teachers teach their students, but just behind them is a system that integrates their work with that of administrators, staff, and parents on behalf of their teaching relationships. Social workers, counselors, and therapists work with their clients, but behind them is a system that integrates their work with a set of administrators, staff, and community members whose jobs entail supporting the creation and process of those caregiving relationships. Nurses, physicians, and other healthcare workers work to heal patients, but behind them are scores of others who foster those healing relationships through their own roles.

All organizations consist, of course, of people whose jobs are designed in theory to interlock and integrate with others on behalf of the organizing mission. However, certain dimensions that render them resilient mark caregiving systems. In these systems, members constantly and successfully struggle to maintain integration in spite of constant pressures to the contrary; they create temporary holding environments with and for one another and they are bound by a set of shared cultural beliefs and practices. In this chapter, I describe and illustrate these dimensions.

Pressing toward integration

A constant press toward integrated efforts marks caregiving systems. Like all organizations, caregiving systems contain a number of splits and divisions – across tasks, functions, departments, and hierarchies – as members organize to attend to different dimensions of their work with clients, patients, students, and various types of careseeker. Hospitals are divided into units and wards, based partly on the various medical problems that patients present. Schools are divided into departments, by subject, or grades. Social service agencies are divided into various functional areas according to which segments of the community – clients, funding organizations, government agencies – members interface with. Organizations divide up internal operations to match the various tasks they need to accomplish. These divisions press members toward dis-integration, that is, toward attending to their immediate interests and demands. Organizations that struggle well to withstand that press, and integrate on behalf of those they serve, create themselves as caregiving systems.

Consider, for example, the workings of a typical hospital. Patients enter the hospital for specific medical conditions and are assigned to particular areas on the basis of the procedures they require – surgery, tests, intensive care, and the like. They are attended to by a variety of organization members, each of whom is responsible for some aspect of the patient's experience: admitting secretaries, nurses, surgeons, physicians representing different medical specialties, social service personnel, various administrators involved in billing, insurance, and community relations. These people pass through the patient's life in the hospital, responsible for different aspects of their experience. The natural press is for them to attend solely to that for which they are responsible: the surgeon considers the patient as, say, "the Tuesday morning gall bladder" or "burst aorta"; the admitting secretary considers only the need to gather the patient's personal information to enter into the records; the nurse focuses solely on the patient's schedule of medication, while the various physicians brought in for consultations or tests frame the patient in terms of their particular specialties.

On the surface, this is exactly what organizational life is like. People specialize in certain tasks and attend to careseekers in ways that enable them to accomplish those tasks efficiently and well. The press, however, is for members to focus so intently on their specific tasks that in the space between them is a void. There is little integration, except for relatively brief transitions – hit-and-run interactions – between members as they hand patients to one another, consult briefly over charts and test results, and schedule the next steps of the patient's journey. What gets lost in the typical hospital is *integration on behalf of the patient*. In hospitals that "struggle well," however, members strive to work together as much as they can. Teams of physicians and nurses are collectively responsible for patients. Hospital staff members invest time with one another in managing transitions, as patients move from surgery to intensive care, or between medical testing rooms, communicating their understandings of what patients are experiencing or need. Hospital administrators look in on patients and inquire about their experiences, and seek to provide hospital staff with the resources necessary to care properly for the patients. Hospital members collaborate with one another, creating an integrated caregiving system.

A number of conditions enable this press toward integration in caregiving organizations. They include the following: the use of the primary task as an integrating mechanism; clearly differentiated roles and authority; and structural interdependence.

Primary task as integrating mechanism

Caregiving systems are anchored by a shared focus on the primary task of the organization. The primary task – defined earlier as that which the organization must perform in order to survive – serves as a touchstone for members who join together to create caregiving systems. Teachers and administrators join around the task of creating meaningful classroom relationships and environments. Social workers, supervisors, administrators, and fundraisers join around the task of serving the specific needs of their clients, just as nurses, physicians, staff, and administrators join around the task of healing patients. Members consistently refer to the primary task; they tether themselves to it, as lifeguards attach themselves to lifelines as they head out toward swimmers struggling in the sea.

This seems patently obvious. If asked, members of caregiving organizations would routinely say that they join around their primary tasks and they would believe it so. It is, however, not always the case, as individuals, groups and units pursue their own interests. When they do so they inevitably fragment those they mean to help. Patients, clients, students, and congregants are seen not as whole people, but as something else altogether: as the "kidney stone in ward 12," the "addict," the "homeless AIDS guy," and other labels that tend to reduce careseekers to some part of who they are. Caregiving systems are marked by members who try to hold onto the fullness of those with whom they work. They do so by collaborating with one another, integrating their work in order to collectively serve the needs of the people who seek their help as teachers, healthcare workers, social workers, and clergy. They integrate in order to maintain a sense of integrated others. When organizations are dis-integrated, they are marked by the loss of the primary task.

Integrity of roles and authority

Integration is also related to how people assume their roles and their authority in relation to one another. When roles have integrity, they are clearly differentiated from one another, and members hold onto them in the face of pressures otherwise. Individuals are clear about their own tasks and how they fit with the tasks of others. They are clear as well about their own authority, defined in terms of the decisions for which they are responsible. People are clear about who participates in what settings and decisions, how they do so, and when they do so. Moreover, they are able to follow those rules. They hold onto their roles, rather than let them go and covertly enact others; they hold onto their appropriate authority, rather than assume that which is not theirs or step away from that which is (Lyth 1988; Rice 1963; Shapiro & Carr 1991). They maintain appropriate boundaries in relation to one another and to careseekers.

Consider, for example, a school. The role of the senior administrator – the principal, headmaster, dean – is to develop and deploy resources, create a vision for the institution, and ensure that appropriate, engaging instructional relationships are being developed on behalf of student learning. The role of the teachers is to create meaningful relationships with their students, collaborate effectively with one another on behalf of their students, and create opportunities for students to learn. The roles of the various staff – secretaries, computer technicians, nurses, janitors – involve supporting the work of the school, through effective operation and maintenance as well as their own relationships with students and one another. Each actor in this setting has certain authority to make and enact certain decisions. Administrators' authority is related to goals, resources, and personnel; teachers' authority is related to that which occurs within their departments and classrooms; staff members' authority is related to that which falls within their particular provinces. In resilient schools, members of each of these groups use their authority in relation to one another and the students in spite of the inevitably difficult, often painful repercussions. They remain within the boundaries of their roles, in spite of the pulls on them – by their colleagues as well as students – to do or be something else altogether.

Structural interdependence

Integration is, finally, a structural matter. While the particular structure of any particular caregiving organization looks quite different depending on its work, it typically involves discrete units, such as departments, teams, and groups organized around specific tasks. The tasks are either related to working with careseekers, such as a radiology department in a hospital, history department in a school, or housing service in a social service agency, or related to internal organizational operations, such as a senior management team in a clinic, a board of directors for a church, or a group of supervisors in a residential treatment center. Most caregiving organizations have such structural arrangements. In resilient organizations these units, as a matter of course, act interdependently. Members do not work in isolation from other units. They do not simply focus on their own tasks but seek to collaborate with other units to meet the needs of careseekers.

For example, consider a community mental health clinic. The clinic is divided into inpatient wards (for acute psychiatric issues) and outpatient treatment centers (for addictions and non-acute mental health issues). The inpatient and outpatient services each contain staff grouped according to profession: psychiatrists, social workers, nurses, and technicians. A director leads each service; a senior member serving as coordinator leads each staff group. The structure of the clinic involves first, the separation of groups and units from one another, and second, their coalescing in larger forums. Separately, each professional staff group within the inpatient and outpatient units meets regularly to examine its work, in relation to the patients and to one another. Staff members also meet regularly as units, in order to examine their work as a unit. The psychiatrists, social workers, and nurses also meet across the boundaries of the inpatient and outpatient units, in order to discuss patients that move between units. The units also coalesce in the context of clinic-wide meetings, in which members from across the organization join together to examine their effectiveness with their clients. They have the opportunity to integrate across the divisions that typically press toward their being split apart in the face of their seemingly disjointed tasks.

This clinic operates as a caregiving system when its members are able to use these various settings as regular opportunities for collaboratively identifying and solving increasingly larger problems in the context of increasingly larger forums. Two characteristics mark this process. First, the *hierarchical* underpinnings of the organization support structural interdependence. Leaders require, model, reward, and reinforce members for working out problems and solutions together, within and across units, rather than leaving unresolved issues at the doorstep of the leaders themselves (Miller 1993). Second, the *boundaries* of each unit, professional group, and hierarchical level allow for both belonging and separation (Alderfer 1980a; Minuchin 1974). Each group meets to work on issues related to the tasks their members share in common. They create boundaries that differentiate them from the rest of the system. Thus, the senior managers work as a group to create visions and systems for accountability rather than slide away from that work, not meet, and let their authority trickle down to other parts of the system. Boundaries are also permeable enough, however, to enable groups to take in and impart information to one another. The psychiatrists meet together to discuss patterns they observe in the patients, using information they have gathered from nurses and social workers, and develop insights that they both use and share with others. Such boundaries allow members to identify with both the work of their specific units and with the organization as a whole.

Holding environments at work

In caregiving systems, members also work with one another in ways that actively generate within one another, and in particular within direct caregivers, the experience of being absorbed, digested, and provided for. Members feel contained and held within the context of their work relations. These systems operate on a simple, powerful principle: caregiving that flows throughout work relationships among organization members maintains a steady flow into careseekers and, not incidentally, an ongoing stream by which to maintain a resilient organization.

This formulation is neither idealistic nor magical. It makes sense both conceptually and practically. In the first chapter I described caregiving organizations as open systems that import, convert, and export materials in order to survive (Rice 1963). Caregivers exist on the boundary of their organiza-tions, interfacing with careseekers. In order to remain at that boundary, and remain effective in their work, they must also be connected in ongoing ways with their organizations. They must ensure they are adequately representing their organizations' missions, current states of resources, and interests. Their organizations must ensure that they are extracting from direct caregivers the information they need to develop and implement strategies that serve organ-izational and community interests. Caregivers and other organization mem-bers must thus maintain connections close enough to enable each to learn from the other. Without such connections, caregivers would drift closer to careseekers, and the organization would lose them and the information they represent. Examples of this abound – teachers identifying more with their students than with one another or their administration, social workers left on their own to serve too many clients without enough supervision – and are considered in more depth in the following chapter.

Theorists frame these connections in various ways. Likert (1967) uses the phrase *system of supportive relationships*, and Lyth (1988) the term *thera-peutic milieu*, to describe social systems in which ongoing social support among members helps to prevent emotional and physical withdrawals. Such patterns create trusting and caring environments that enable organizations to combat burnout (Pines & Aronson 1988). They enable organization members to be, as Lyth (1988: 253) noted, "Contained in a system of meaningful attachments." Lyth's phrasing is important here. Organization members may be contained. This occurs, she suggests, in the context of a system of attach-ments. In resilient caregiving organizations, this occurs as a matter of course. Members routinely and consistently inquire about and attend to others, validate and empathize with them, support and show compassion for them. Such acts require neither extensive personal relationships nor therapeutic, counseling relationships. They are part of, rather than separate from, work interactions. They denote an attention to the person of the other, a valuing of the other's self and experiences.

In practice, this is a constant series of calibrations: movements toward (i.e., inquiries into experiences, attentive listening, provision of resources), and movements away from others, enabling people to go off and do their work. A supervisor at a mental health clinic sits with a social worker and helps him understand his increasing resentment of a client. A school administrator meets with a committee of teachers having difficulty develop-ing a new curriculum, and after listening to their experiences, helps them identify the sources of difficulty and several strategies for moving ahead. A board member helps a clergy member examine his mounting frustration with a group of congregants who are pressing for radical change. A hospital administrator listens carefully to the complaints of nurses struggling to adapt to a new technology and offers to design, with their help, a training session.

These acts are, in some ways, simply examples of good management and leadership. They are performed, however, in ways that leave caregivers and other members feeling valued, listened to, and joined rather than left alone – the core acts of being cared for. Organization members come together, across roles, and create temporary holding environments at work (Kahn 2001). In so doing, they replenish the stores of care that flow out toward careseekers, through the vessels of the caregivers. Thus they create systems of attachments that in turn create resiliency throughout the organization, as though inflating its contours with a layer of buoyancy. When members are laid low by the daily traumas or explosive crises that mark their work lives, their falls are cushioned by the nature of their attachments with one another. Their organizations provide an "arms-around experience" (Josselson 1992). They are held fast.

Flows of supervision

Resilient organizations are also characterized by flows of supervision that infiltrate both hierarchical and peer settings. At each level of the resilient organization, members supervise others. Just as direct caregivers work to absorb, digest, and work with the experiences of careseekers, members do so in relation to those for whom they are responsible. Supervision within resilient organizations parallels the process of providing care to careseekers: attending to others in ways that leave them feeling valued and cared for. Effective supervisors enable those they supervise to feel contained. They empathically acknowledge them and help them gain perspective. In short, they provide holding. The principle here is simply this: providing people with the regular experience of being held enables them to do the same for others. Caring for others fills them up with caring, which they then have available to pass on.

This is crucial for caregivers, of course. Therapists, childcare workers, social workers, and others who work directly with mental health receive supervision, typically from senior members of their fields. In other resilient caregiving organizations, teachers are supervised by headteachers or administrators, nurses by nurse managers or directors, physicians by unit chiefs or administrators. In regular contact, supervisors enable staff to share their experiences, work through that which disturbs them, and develop and implement effective actions. They create temporary holding environments, which close around caregivers and then reopen, enabling them to emerge with heightened capacities to engage their work.

Similarly, front-line supervisors have their own settings in which they receive that which they provide to caregivers. Hospital administrators supervise department heads. Departmental coordinators in treatment centers supervise the supervisors of the staff workers. School vice-principals and assistant deans supervise department heads and chairpersons. Operating officers in social service agencies supervise program directors. In turn, senior managers – executive directors, principals, deans, and chief executive officers – supervise their own subordinates, the middle managers on whom they depend to manage the discrete operations of their organizations. The most senior executives seek their own supervision, outside the boundaries of their organizations: they work with consultants, avail themselves of board members, or seek supervision with peers and mentors from other organizations.

The resilient caregiving organization is marked by this flow of supervision down through the hierarchy. Pools of caring are created at each level, and spill over like waterfalls down the organization, finally depositing in streams of careseekers. There are eddies as well, where members within hierarchical groups sustain one another with various forms of peer supervision. Social workers, therapists, physicians, nurses, teachers, and childcare workers meet regularly without supervisors, working through cases with one another. They vent, share information, provide support, and organize for change. Similar settings are created at other levels, albeit with different purposes. Front-line supervisors meet to discuss patterns of staffing, while middle managers meet in order to examine how to integrate their operations more effectively. Senior management teams meet to develop strategy that will enable them to effectively serve the needs of changing markets.

While the tasks of these meetings differ, what occurs within them is, in the context of resilient organizations, strikingly similar to that which occurs in supervision settings. Members attend closely to one another, provide feedback and perspective, and work on shared projects collaboratively. They leave one another feeling more rather than less valued.

Resilient cultures

Resilience in caregiving organizations is strengthened by a set of shared, often unspoken beliefs among members. These beliefs guide members, directing them toward certain types of behavior in various types of situation. They become woven into the cultures of organizations, where they exist as mostly unquestioned assumptions among members (Schein 1999). As such, they provide instinctive answers to questions that routinely confront members. In caregiving organizations such questions are at the core of members' experiences: *What do we do when we are stressed, verging on overwhelmed? How are we supposed to feel and think at those times? How are we supposed to work with and be with one another? How do we use our personal selves in the context of our work?* These and similarly fundamental questions are answered in particular ways in resilient caregiving organizations. The answers are in the form of three types of belief that are made visible through the behaviors of members. These beliefs hold members together; they are a cultural skin that binds them in the face of both daily stress and extraordinary events.

The strength of work relationships

A primary belief at the heart of a resilient organization culture is that members move toward rather than away from one another when they experience stress and anxiety. Members and leaders have a core conviction that they must band together, within and across the various groups that mark their organization, if they are to thrive individually and collectively. They assume that they are best able to find shelter and strength in their work relations with one another. At a deeper, unarticulated level, they believe that their relations are, ultimately, the source of power, faith, love, and hope – the necessary ingredients to remain alive and effective in the work of teaching, healing, ministering to, and in other ways caring for others. They believe, and thus enact, the idea that resilience is created and found in the space between them, in the work relationships that they create and maintain.

This belief is enacted both in how people go about their daily work together and how they instinctively react to troubling situations. In resilient organizations, members place primary importance on clear communication processes. Leaders and members work hard to share information with one another, even in the context of authority structures that make it more difficult for them to communicate openly. They make time to meet and clarify situations rather than rush to respond without a complex understanding of what they are trying to do and why. They listen actively to one another. They have a history of collaborative problem-solving. They approach problems together, diagnosing their causes and developing solutions. They disagree, of course, and at various times struggle to influence one another, negotiating interests and resolutions. They do so, however, in the context of valuing their work relationships, trusting that any solution that sacrifices those relationships will not be acceptable.

Members are thus resilient because of their belief that they cannot thrive outside their relations with one another. They turn together toward stress and trauma rather than turn upon one another. The school administrators and teachers meeting after the knife incident struggle with possible solutions. They go back and forth about whether to install metal detectors or security officers and discuss the implications for their ability to create trusting relations with students. They state their cases passionately. They ask probing questions, eliciting information and perceptions. They listen closely to one another, seeking understanding. They work toward a solution, understanding that it will be imperfect like all solutions but that they must each assume responsibility for helping to implement it. They leave their meetings feeling that they have worked together as well as they might. They leave feeling joined with rather than set apart from others, and that whatever occurs in the wake of their decision, they are in it together. At the heart of resilience is this sense of *being in it together*, of members knowing that they will not have to face difficulties by themselves.

The importance of emotional life

A second belief central to resilience is that beneath people's daily routines of meetings, talking on phones, writing memos and other routines there is another sort of reality worth attending to: the emotions that members experience while working with careseekers and one another. I noted earlier that members, particularly caregivers, might feel quite a lot in the course of their work. They may be filled up with careseekers' emotions as a byproduct of taking in and absorbing careseekers. They may have emotional reactions of their own, triggered by their work. In resilient caregiving organizations these emotions are respected, in the way that sailors respect the open sea: as powerful and deep, mysterious and important, able to carry them along or inflict significant damage upon them, and not to be taken lightly. Members and leaders believe that emotions – theirs and careseekers' – offer valuable information about their work with careseekers and with one another. They believe that attending to emotions enables them to create the relationships they need to survive in the work.

This belief is enacted in how people work with emotions on a daily basis. They engage in relatively open emotional expression. They tell one another when they are upset or saddened by a certain event or case. They express their joy to one another. They tolerate rather than turn away from difficult emotions triggered in their work with one another or with their students, patients, clients, or congregants. They do this as part of their routine interactions, checking in with one another whenever they meet. They also do this when it is most difficult and most important to do so, when painful affect is triggered by particular events. At those moments people are often likely to avoid contact, pushing away from one another in order to push away the affect itself. In resilient organizations they move toward one another rather than withdraw or erect barriers against their colleagues. They do so in order to help themselves and others get out from under the weight of pressing emotions. They seek to learn the meaning of those emotions, for themselves and their work with others.

Consider the example of a residential treatment center whose members are trying to understand an outbreak of violence by their adolescent clients. Staff members are being sworn at, hit, and spat upon. Some staff members are angry and upset, others frightened, and still others saddened by the events. Their own work relationships are being disturbed; as some staff react to the clients with discipline and others react with nurturance, each becomes upset with the others' strategies. In passing hallway conversations, staff members tell one another of their frustrations with their clients and agree that they need to meet and discuss the situation more fully. A supervisor arranges a meeting at the end of the shift. Staff members talk more fully about their anger at the clients and at one another. They speak of their confusion about the causes of the violence, and of their fears for their physical safety. They tell stories about being attacked and how it felt. Then they stop telling stories and reflect on why they are so angry, upset, and frightened. They reflect well enough to decode the messages being sent to them by their clients – how they are angry and afraid, and what this might refer to. It turns out to be a situation in which a new overnight worker had supplied drugs to a client, which, once known among the other clients, upset their sense of safety and boundaries. They reacted with violence, not knowing how else to communicate their anger and fear. The communication was received and acted upon, due in no small measure to the residential staff's abilities to share and examine their emotions.

This process is predicated on the shared belief that emotions, in oneself or within others, are important to attend to, both as a source of data and for effective working relationships. In resilient organizations, members tell stories that keep emotions as central, not peripheral or absent. They reflect on them and what they might mean. They adopt what Shapiro and Carr (1991) call "the interpretive stance": the examination of one's experiences and emotions for what they might reveal about one's role and task. When members engage in this practice together, they seek to create a shared understanding of events, situations, and experiences. They believe that the different emotions that have been located in them, by careseekers and one another, need to be unpacked and examined for what they suggest about their work. Some residential staff were angry, others sad; some reacted punitively, some with nurturance. Believing that all of these emotions and reactions were valid, staff members were able to examine them as *information*. They did not blame or personally attack one another; nor did they scapegoat particular staff members or clients. They joined rather than split apart from one another. They were enabled by rather than disabled from their work relations. And their emotional reactions were validated and normalized by one another, leaving them cleared of emotions that might otherwise render them unable to absorb others.

The world as manageable

The third belief associated with resilience is that organizational life is manageable, comprehensible and meaningful. Organization members believe that adversity can be overcome, and indeed, is necessary to strengthen people. When people believe that they have some control over events in their world – that what they do will make a difference, that their influence is real and predictable – they are more likely to actually try and shape events positively. Seligman (1998) refers to this phenomenon as "learned optimism." Resilient individuals are noteworthy for their sense of optimism. They believe that they can influence events, that they are not simply helpless or powerless. Organizational cultures may be similarly characterized, to the extent that their members share a powerful, often unspoken belief in their collective abilities to exert influence, render their environments meaningful, and manage that which comes their way.

This belief is evident in both how organization members approach their work and the stories they tell of their work experiences. Adverse situations are approached not with fear and trepidation but as opportunities to learn and grow. People do not pretend that difficult situations are not difficult. Rather, they appreciate the difficulty but assume that they have, or can find, the resources and abilities to manage the situations. They assume that they can resolve them in ways that leave their work and themselves intact. Simply put, they believe that they can handle such situations, and, buoyed by that belief, they do so. Members and leaders then tell and retell stories that make clear that they have met and overcome adversity. They make sense of the adversity, rendering it comprehensive and meaningful. In telling stories of events, they communicate the larger story of meeting challenges, overcoming adversity, and becoming the stronger for it. They tell and retell the story of their own resilience and in doing so they become increasingly resilient.

Take, for example, how a social service agency deals with a sudden rise in social workers' absenteeism and turnover. Half of the agency's social workers have left over the course of a year, with others considering the same. The agency's executive director gathers together the supervisors and leads a series of unflinchingly candid conversations about the nature of the jobs that social workers are being asked to do. They discover together that the context of their work has shifted: that the closing of public and private psychiatric facilities has increased the acuity of the mental illnesses that their social workers are working with on a daily basis, while the support systems in place for those workers have not shifted accordingly. They reflect together on what they need to do to create an appropriate support system. Their conversations are marked by curiosity, a sense of wanting to explore and understand the situation they and their social workers find themselves in. They see the problem as simply that – a problem needing to be openly examined and solved, rather than as a situation that is in some fashion unmanageable and from which they need to hide.

In such instances resilience is both enacted and created by members' shared belief that they can survive and learn from whatever they discover in the course of examining and solving problems. The belief leads to the reality: members assume that they can handle adversity and make it manageable, and it becomes so. The reality in turn reinforces the belief: members overcome adversity and come to believe that their world is manageable. This is the underlying, mutually reinforcing cycle of resilience; it is a self-fulfilling prophecy, writ large at the level of the organization.

The creation of capacity

Resilient organizations are marked by such mutually reinforcing cycles. Through structures that press them toward integration, flows of supervision and caring behaviors, and shared beliefs around integration, members move toward one another. They work in the shelter of one another. This enables them to withstand both the daily press of their work and the episodic jolts that threaten to disrupt their work. They become resilient, able to absorb a great deal without being paralyzed or disrupted. The experience of such resilience – of surviving, even thriving, in the face of what is often quite difficult work – in turn reinforces enabling structures, processes, and beliefs. The cycle continues, uninterrupted, as long as organization members continue to move toward one another, stay the course of their work together, and experience themselves as effective. With such cycles, the question often arises as to how they came into being. How do resilient organizations set in motion that which makes and keeps them so? Schein (1999), in his analysis of organizational cultures, offers a likely scenario. He suggests that organizational cultures – and the structures, processes and norms that mark them – develop through a process of trial and error. People, through acts of leadership, organize themselves in ways they hope will prove successful. They create certain organizational arrangements and ways of working with one another and their clients or customers. When they find arrangements that are demonstrably effective, indicating that they will survive as organizations, they begin to solidify those arrangements. Over time those arrangements, reinforced through continued success, become the accepted, often unquestioned way by which members function. They become *cultures*. Resilient caregiving organizations thus develop as they do because leaders and members discovered that by joining together through integrating structures, relationships and beliefs, they were able to sustain themselves and their careseekers. They were rewarded by that which made them resilient, which made them seek to be more so.

These cycles both create and enlarge the capacities of caregiving organization members to engage in their work. The notion of capacity is an important one. The word itself, derived from the Latin *capere*, means "to take, hold, contain." It has various common usages and I draw upon several here. First, it refers to the power that individuals (and thus their organizations) have to receive or contain others, i.e., their ability to take into "storage" a certain amount of work, affect, and other people, much like the volume capacity of batteries. Second, it refers to productive output, like the capability of manufacturing plants, i.e., members' collective capability to serve others. Capacity thus refers to the end points of what defines open systems, which operate by taking in and transforming inputs (via processes collectively termed "throughput") into outputs aligned with the guiding, primary task of the organization (Rice 1963). In resilient caregiving organizations, people engage in "throughput" processes in ways that enhance their capacities to absorb and contain others (take input) and meet their needs (produce output).

In practice this means that when people create caregiving *systems*, they generate a capacity to absorb and work with others. They continuously clear space to take in others and work with them without being so filled up that they need to shut down, emotionally or cognitively, with no available space. Nurses working with a ward of hepatitis C patients make time to help one another talk about and cope with setbacks in their patients' progress. Teachers and administrators at a public high school together create a program for parents in the community to learn about dealing with adolescents. Social workers and their supervisors meet regularly as a group to work through the implications of reduced funding for their programs and services, examining the impact on their relations with clients and one another and developing strategies for improving the lives of both. Nurses, aides, and physicians staffing a psychiatric treatment center in which a patient recently committed suicide hold open staff meetings through which to examine the implications of that act for themselves and their patients. Childcare workers at a residential treatment center work with staff therapists to design and implement a social skills program for their clients. Clergy and administrative staff at a church work together with a consultant to examine causes and solutions related to a dwindling population of congregants.

In such settings, resilience is created when members move toward one another to engage themselves and their work, supported by a set of integrating structures and practices, caring relations with one another, and beliefs in the efficacy of their work together. Working together enlarges members' capacities. Sharing experiences and acknowledging anxiety and painful affect helps to clear direct caregivers of difficult emotions soaked up from others or triggered by the work. By collaborating across various divides of function, role, and hierarchy, they engage problems rationally and support one another. By creating temporary holding environments with one another, they fill one another up with experiences of being cared for, attended to, and valued. They store those experiences, like holding tanks, and draw them down in the course of delivering care to patients, clients, students, congregants. Their capacities for storage, and for delivery, are enhanced by how they work together.

Such is the resilient caregiving organization. It is marked by flows of caregiving, which look different in particular types of organization and relationship but whose underlying action is the same. There are many ways in which these systems are disrupted. In the next chapter I examine the nature and causes of such disruptions and their implications for caregivers and careseekers alike.

Chapter 4

System breakdowns

A lack of resilience within caregiving organizations presents itself in particular ways. An inpatient mental health clinic is marked by struggles for control between staff nurses and attending psychiatrists. The administrators of a welfare agency are frustrated by the staff's inability to independently solve problems. The government agency charged with protecting children loses a stream of social workers and therapists. Teachers and administrators of a private school remain locked in conflict over how to involve parents in the life of the school. Religious services and programs are badly attended by the members of a congregation whose leaders have been unable to develop a vision for their institution. Nurses and physicians staffing the emergency room of a city hospital have difficulty moving patients out of the unit, stymied by their inability to communicate effectively with other hospital admitting units. A residential treatment center for adolescents is divided into units whose directors do not easily or usefully share resources, ideas, and programs. When these and similar dilemmas present themselves and members cannot as a matter of course resolve them, the organization has a problem with resilience.

At a deeper level, the caregiving organization itself has broken down. It is less a system of caregiving than a series of disconnected units that have little capacity to draw upon one another in the service of the organization's primary task. If the metaphor of the resilient organization is that of a constant flow – of energy, caring, support, emotional and practical resources – among members and with careseekers, then the metaphor of the caregiving organization without resilience is that of blockages, of dams and channels and dead-ends that isolate individuals and groups from one another. Such a situation manifests itself in reasonably familiar ways. Caregivers burn out and withdraw from careseekers. Organization departments and units are at odds; senior administrators are unavailable, too intrusive, or too embattled; middle managers and supervisors are paralyzed, unable to implement strategy or support caregivers, or they are too active, unable to let others act autonomously. Caregivers are too overwhelmed or disempowered to seek support from one another or to demand it from their supervisors. While not often understood as such, these are system breakdowns.

Such breakdowns are not accidental. Nor are they developed on purpose. They exist in a rather more complicated place, beneath the conscious surface understandings of organization members. System breakdowns that do not get resolved by the best efforts of members follow an unconscious, underlying logic that holds them in place. Patterns of behavior and interaction that isolate people from one another, or drive them toward conflict rather than collaboration, or keep them at odds with those they ostensibly serve, are not simply a matter of organizational oversight or incompetence. Rather, they often meet unconscious, irrational but nonetheless important needs of some or all organization members. If dysfunctional patterns did not serve people's needs they would as a matter of course be identified, fixed, and extinguished. Members would organize and rise up in protest, withhold support for initiatives, or turn away from rather than reinforce people's inappropriate behaviors. If members do not respond in such ways it is because they must *want* – at some level – irrational practices to continue.

This follows a psychological premise: when people are unwilling or unable to change behaviors that are clearly irrational, given the goals they articulate, it is often because unconscious, irrational needs are holding sway. Organizations work the same way. They too act in seemingly irrational ways, given their ostensible goals. Their breakdowns may often be traced to irrational purposes that members have collectively, unconsciously substituted for organizational goals. In this chapter I describe the underlying logic of breakdown in caregiving systems, showing how it manifests itself in various ways, toward various ends, and with various consequences.

The underlying logic of system breakdowns

Dysfunctional patterns of organizational behavior that are tolerated rather than extinguished are held in place because they defend members against anxiety. System breakdowns often begin in response to organization members' desires to move away from the powerful, primitive feelings that get evoked and deposited within them. Because of their identifications with careseekers, they might feel pity, fear, sorrow, or depression; revulsion, despair, inadequate, or helpless; attracted, angry, or violent. This holds true not simply for direct caregivers but for other members – administrators, staff, support personnel – as well. Such reactions are not easy to experience. They are even more difficult to tolerate when one must at the same time get work done. People often wish to move away from a conscious experience of such reactions and the anxiety they trigger. They do so through the time-honored tradition of psychological defense mechanisms. "Insofar as feelings cannot be worked with personally or institutionally," writes Lyth (1988: 230), "they are likely to be dealt with by the development of defences against them."

People trying to rid themselves of distress by pushing away the conscious experience of pain and anxiety often seek the same sort of relief as careseekers:

they too wish to push away, export, or in other ways distance themselves from the source of their distress. Unlike careseekers, however, members of caregiving organizations may be supported in their defensive endeavors by one another and by their institutions. Indeed, they may become part of an *institutional defense system* that has as its aim the protection of part or the whole of the organization itself from seemingly destabilizing anxiety.

This formulation has its roots in the work of Wilfred Bion (1961). Bion developed the idea that groups may be understood at two levels of analysis. They are sophisticated work groups, working on overt tasks. They are also what Bion termed "basic groups," acting upon covert basic assumptions that enable members to avoid work on their primary task. Bion found that when a group's primary task represented a reality that was painful or caused psychological conflict within or between members, they would unconsciously direct their behaviors toward reducing the anxiety and conflict. Members would take the group off course, pursuing tangents, discussing trivial matters, creating skirmishes that enabled group members to avoid confronting the conflicts related to the primary task. They avoided their primary tasks. In doing so they lost touch with reality and its demands. They lost their ability to work, which necessarily involves tolerating frustration, facing reality, recognizing differences among group members, and learning from experience (Stokes 1994). The basic assumption group acts as if to work directly on the primary task would be to risk its psychological survival.

Consider, for example, a group of teachers whose school had recently been subject to drastic cuts related to the restructuring of the local educational system (adapted from Roberts 1994b). The school was known for innovative programs in the areas of work experience and career counseling, which were threatened by the cuts. The teachers responded by withdrawing from their students and from one another. Their meetings became exercises in avoidance: they focused on incidental items, like the colors of the commencement banner; they wasted entire sessions blaming the local superintendent; they let one senior teacher lead them in a pointless effort to redesign a recently developed language curriculum. They thus avoided their anxiety about what would now happen to their students, given the high local unemployment and relative poverty. In defending against the experience and expression of that anxiety the teachers were unable to act in ways that might have proven useful: organize campaigns for students and families, engage the local media, or examine how they might cut less necessary programs to fund those they felt were most important for their students. Their need to defend themselves psychologically prevented them from acting as a sophisticated work group.

Bion's (1961) work offers a compelling framework for understanding such stubbornly irrational patterns. Tavistock Institute theorists applied this framework to an analysis of various organizations (see Jacques 1974; Lyth 1988; Miller 1993; Rice 1963). They demonstrated that members defend against collective anxiety by instituting dysfunctional ways of relating and working together. Jacques (1974) described how social systems supported individuals' psychological defenses to ward off anxiety, operating in ways that enabled them to avoid certain internal conflicts. The covert actions of such social defense mechanisms revealed themselves in their persistent effects. "Behavior that is inadequately related to reality," Miller (1993: 39) writes, "and that the people concerned would themselves acknowledge in other circumstances to be irrational or abnormal, is *prima facie* evidence of the presence of anxiety." Feelings of anxiety are at the root of distorted or alienated relationships at work, which warp people's collective capacity to accomplish primary tasks (Hirschhorn 1988). Such diminishment of capacities lies at the heart of defense mechanisms that sap the resilience of caregiving organizations.

Social defenses

Institutional or social defenses can be healthy, enabling people to cope with stress (Halton 1994). They may also be unhealthy, like individual defenses, when they distance organization members from reality, hinder their work, damage them in some fashion, and prevent their adapting to changing circumstances (Skogstad 2000). The classic study of social defenses by Lyth (1988) revealed the depth to which their dysfunctionality was embedded in an organization's structure, systems, and culture. Her study of a nursing service of a teaching hospital revealed the widespread use of certain defenses against the anxiety related to working with diseased patients. Individual nurses performed specific tasks (e.g., bed-making, washing) for many patients, thus restricting contact with any one patient. Patients were discussed as bed numbers or diseases rather than by name, and were treated according to the disease category into which they fell. Nurses moved throughout the unit on their shifts, limiting their abilities to attach to specific patients. They were taught to not care about or get involved with patients. They routinely denied disturbing feelings. They rushed about the unit, engaging routinely in pressured activity that provided little time for intimate contact with patients, or for that matter with one another.

The nurses' excessive movements throughout the unit trained them to remain disconnected from their patients. They were unable to form meaningful attachments in which powerful, disturbing feelings might have been evoked. The social defenses worked by eliminating situations, events, tasks, activities, and relationships that caused anxiety. Nurses avoided getting close to the suffering and death of their patients by not allowing themselves – or being allowed by their unit's formal structure and informal norms – to get close to particular patients. This profoundly shaped nurses' relationships with patients. They were unable to perceive and work with them as whole people. Patients were taken in and worked with as fragmented parts: they were specific diseases, operations, or conditions, framed in terms of specific tasks rather than as people who were suffering physically and emotionally. As a result, the nurses themselves became fragmented. Unable to attach to individual patients and work with their humanness – their suffering, hopes, fears – the nurses were left without a place for their own complex humanness. They walled off the parts of themselves that sought expression in contact with their patients. Unable to invest their whole selves in their work they left parts of those selves out of their work (Kahn 1992). They became alienated in and from their work, i.e., parts of their selves were alien to them when they were at work.

Lyth (1988) further identified how the social defenses in the nursing service shaped relationships among the nurses themselves. A split developed between the junior and senior nurses in the service. The senior nurses were identified as the disciplinarians, focused on maintaining separation from patients. The junior nurses were identified as irresponsible, unable to manage the complexity of their work tasks. This split represented an unconscious collusion. The nurses joined together, at a deep and unarticulated level, to avoid the pain and anxiety related to the difficulty of their work. They created between the two groups interpersonal and intergroup conflicts, between those who seemed too harsh and those who seemed too incompetent. This took the place of a more difficult intrapsychic conflict that existed within each of them: their desire to protect themselves by distancing from patients, versus their sense of inadequacy at not being able to engage with patients in ways that would alleviate suffering. The nurses sought to evade this intrapsychic conflict by colluding to have different groupings – senior and junior – carry the different sides. They then isolated the groups from one another: each side kept itself apart from the other, on the basis of a series of projected beliefs about the other ("harsh," "slow learner"). By maintaining such projections they ensured that the split would remain. Their internal conflicts became located outside themselves.

The nursing service study revealed the classic characteristics of social defenses. Individuals use formal organizational structures, such as nursing rotations, and informal norms, such as discussing patients as diseases, to help evade anxiety. They also use relatively primitive psychic defenses such as avoidance, denial, splitting, and projection. The defenses are institutionalized, supported by the routine structures, systems and processes of organizational life. People thus create what Lyth (1988) characterizes as anti-therapeutic systems of interpersonal relationships with patients and with one another. Relationships with careseekers are overly bounded and circumscribed. They are taken care *of*, technically, but not necessarily cared *for*. Relationships among staff members are similarly circumscribed. Communication is partial rather than full as members become identified with smaller sub-groups, formal and informal, which they maintain through various projections about "others." The primary caregiving task is thus lost; in its place is the task of maintaining social defenses against anxiety.

Social defenses are characterized by the evasion of anxiety but do little to modify and reduce it. The collusive relationships that staff members create with one another are likely to be anti-supportive (Lyth 1988). Locked within perceptions of one another that help maintain social defenses, caregiving organization members are unable to create the types of holding relationships with one another that would enable them to contain the anxiety generated by their primary tasks. Nor is the organization itself able to do so. As Lyth (1988: 63) writes, "Little attempt is made positively to help the individual confront the anxiety-provoking experiences, and by so doing, to develop her capacity to tolerate and deal more effectively with the anxiety." As a result, caregiving organization members are left with secondary anxieties generated by social defenses. They are relatively isolated from one another. They are alienated from themselves. They receive little satisfaction from their work with others, with whom they have few meaningfully human relations. They feel distanced from rather than attached to others at work. In avoiding the emotions and anxiety of their primary tasks, they develop other psychic discomforts.

Anti-task boundaries

The social defenses that characterize some caregiving units and organizations undermine their resilience in a very particular way: they disrupt the boundaries through which workers are defined as members of the same system. Resilience depends on members joining together, on integrating across units for purposes of collaboration and support. Social defenses are dis-integrating mechanisms. They create and propagate inappropriate boundaries. In some instances, boundaries become too rigid; they become what Alderfer (1980a) describes as "over-bounded" or what Minuchin (1974) refers to as "disengaged." The boundary between supervisors and primary caregivers, for example, might become so tight that the former are too distant to provide support while the latter are too untrusting to provide crucial information about careseekers. In other instances, boundaries become too loose; they become "under-bounded" (Alderfer 1980a) or "enmeshed" (Minuchin 1974). In the example above, the supervisors and their managers might merge into one group, and in so doing lose the separate functions of administrative and clinical oversight.

Inappropriate boundaries routinely serve social defenses. The lack of appropriate boundaries may enable non-caregivers to distance themselves from the caregivers and whatever disturbing emotions or anxieties they are feared to have soaked up. In the example above, the supervisors are brought into the shelter of the administrative boundary. They step away from their supervisory roles. The organization more generally loses its ability to absorb and contain careseekers. It becomes dis-integrated. The boundaries disrupt integration across groups (supervisors and caregivers); they undermine the integrity of the necessary separation between groups (administrators and supervisors). The organization cannot contain members within a shared boundary, without which members cannot have the sense that they are all working on the same primary task. They cannot move toward one another, as separate but related units, for support and collaborative work. They move too far away from or too close to one another, disrupting their ability to become resilient through their work relationships. They live within anti-task boundaries (Lyth 1988; Roberts 1994b) that enable members to use their relationships to avoid anxiety related to their primary tasks.

Driving this disruption is the action of institutional splitting and projection. Klein (1959) described splitting as the process of dividing feelings into differentiated elements, as when a child feeling both love and rage toward her mother splits her mother-image into good and bad. Projection is when some of those feelings are located in others rather than in oneself, as when the child acts as if it is her brother who really believes that her mother is bad and she who believes her mother is good. Social defenses are institutional versions of splitting and projecting. People act as if some feelings are located only in certain segments of a group or organization, leaving other segments free to contain other emotions (Lyth 1988; Obholzer & Roberts 1994). In the nursing service, the junior nurses felt routinely inadequate and guilty, enabling the senior nurses to feel competent and angry. This institutional split replaced the nurses' intrapsychic conflict between feeling at once inadequate and competent, sad and angry. These are difficult emotions to experience simultaneously. They tend to arouse anxiety since the opposing feelings cannot be easily resolved. The social defenses in the nursing service created a way for the nurses to evade that particular anxiety.

Social defenses are thus typically marked by some form of scapegoating, in which one part of a system is used by other parts to contain anxiety (Bion 1961; Hirschhorn 1988; Lyth 1988; Wells 1985). Scapegoating is the symbolic term for what was, in biblical times, a literal process: annually, Hebrews would symbolically cast their sins on a goat and exile it to the desert, ridding the community of its evil. The irrational processes that occur in social defenses are somewhat more complicated, and depend on people's tendencies toward splitting and projecting. They also depend on the fault lines that exist beneath the surface of caregiving organizations.

Organizational fault lines

Social defenses and the system breakdowns they engender operate by exploiting and heightening the divisions that naturally mark caregiving organizations. Caregiving organizations contain various divisions – groups, functions, departments, and hierarchies – that enable members to attend to the various sub-tasks of their work with careseekers. These divisions facilitate work getting done, as members divide the labor and attend to specific pieces of the work of the organization. In resilient organizations these specific pieces are brought together, creating integrated caregiving systems. In less resilient organizations the pieces remain separate, individually or in clumps. The caregiving system is fragmented. The divisions that are so useful for performing specific pieces of the larger work of the organization jut out; they do not fall back easily into place but rather become for their members their primary organizations. They are separated from one another, like pieces of a landmass that once suffered a quake and split apart, forming an archipelago of islands large and small.

The normal divisions of an organization are thus joined on the surface but in danger of being split apart along the fault lines lying beneath the surface. In resilient organizations the fault lines are not so prominent. They are not so pronounced as to have been activated by a quake or its aftershocks; or, if activated, they have gradually receded. As described earlier, there is a fair amount of strain that buffets members of caregiving organizations, through the routine action of their work with others and in the traumatic episodes that may erupt at work. In less resilient organizations, members try to evade the strain. They retreat to their own groupings, sealing themselves off from those whom they perceive as "others." The fault lines split the surface, rending it into bits and pieces, each containing a clutch of members who have become separated from other groups. The landscape has altered. Where there might have been relatively flat surfaces over which would flow resources, support, and information, there are jutting walls, gaping holes, and rising mounds of earth. As Halton (1994: 15) notes, "The gaps between departments or professions are available to be filled with many different emotions – denigration, competition, hatred, prejudice, paranoia." This makes impossible the flow of holding and supervision that mark resilient organizations. It makes impossible a *system* whereby members are joined together, meaningfully attached to one another, backing one another up in their struggle to perform their primary task. Institutional divisions beget splits; splits beget system breakdowns.

These breakdowns are driven by organization members seeking refuge in the make-believe. They unconsciously collude to stage plays, casting one another into roles along the fault lines marking the structural divisions between organizational groupings to drive the action. These plays offer refuge. They enable members to retreat from the anxiety generated by the task. Like anxious children, members may regress to the point where they create a more psychically tolerable world in which to act and over which to exert control. A type of make-believe that is difficult to spot thus marks social defenses. Members stage plays of which they are often unaware, for the very specific purpose of helping them avoid *being* aware of that which they feel they cannot tolerate. The specific characters and plots of these plays are often drawn from the populations of careseekers with whom the organization works. Childcare workers act out against one another in ways that echo those of their youth, while staff at an alcoholic treatment facility become abjectly dependent and manipulative toward their leaders just as their clients do toward them.

These unconscious mirrorings are driven by projective identifications, in which careseekers' emotions are deposited into members of caregiving organizations. Members then have their own counter-transferential reactions. In resilient organizations they work through these reactions, in formal (supervisory) and informal (colleagues) holding relationships. In less resilient organizations, members have no such places. They may leave because they cannot tolerate the tensions or anxieties. Or they may try to act as if those reactions do not exist. They too then engage in projective identifications with one another, to rid them of what feels too painful (Moylan 1994). To do this they stage plays. They cast others into roles and project upon them that which they do not wish to hold within themselves.

This process depends on a number of conditions. First, members do not become consciously aware of their participation in this process; insight and reflection weaken the hold of social defenses. Second, members define parts of the organization, including careseekers, as "other" in order to have receptacles to contain their projections. Third, members stay in some relation to the "other" in order to sustain the ongoing process of projective identification. If the "other" was gone, people would themselves have to hold onto emotions and tensions they have tried to evade. Given these three factors, systemic breakdowns are characterized by a particular dynamic: people are unable to reflect together on their patterns of behavior and the functions those patterns truly serve, yet they remain yoked together across various divisions in routinely unhelpful ways that they cannot seem to halt.

Primary splits

Particular types of split weaken the resilience of caregiving organizations in particular ways. In this section of the chapter I illustrate the primary types of organizational split used in the service of social defenses.

Hierarchical splits

Caregiving organizations with hierarchical splits are marked by relatively impermeable boundaries between hierarchical groups. Senior administrators are disconnected from caregivers and those they serve. Supervisors, department heads, and other middle managers occupy the space in between. Each group is isolated from the others. They have enough contact to maintain various projections about one another that impede their collaboration. These projections are often aligned along two primary dimensions: care versus control, and cognitive versus emotional. Senior administrators often anchor the controlling, thinking end of the continua; they are perceived as distant, controlling, quantitative, and calculating. Caregivers anchor the caring, feeling end of the continua; they are perceived as overly nurturing, subjective, qualitative, and emotional. Both sides struggle to co-opt the middle layer of supervisors and administrators, who typically slide up or down in their allegiances rather than hold onto their bridging roles (Oshry 1999).

Consider a social services residential unit for children removed from their families for their own safety (Roberts 1994a). The staff's task involved preparing the children for their eventual return to family life. Staff focused their efforts on creating a secure, home-like place for the children, which made it difficult for them to move back to their homes or foster homes. The staff resisted their manager's attempts to get them back to the organization's primary task, i.e., enabling the children's return to their communities. As Roberts (1994a: 113) writes, "Staff were very suspicious and distrustful of the manager, casting him in the role of a 'bad parent' who was too preoccupied with his own concerns to have the children's best interests at heart."

Much is illustrated by this brief example. The split between the senior manager and the residential staff is marked by a too-rigid boundary: the staff create what Roberts (1994a: 113) terms a "dysfunctionally strong boundary around the child/worker pair." They over-identify with the children and under-identify with the agency's administration. They maintain that split by a set of projections. Residential staff members believe that they are the children's protectors, and that the administrators are dangerous. The social defense in play here requires the staff to act as if they are the ones who care, while their manager is cold to the unmet needs of their charges (and, presumably, to their needs as well). The staff and leaders stage a play whose plot mirrors the projected wishes of the children themselves: to be rescued from the "bad parent" by those willing and able to love them as they wish to be loved.

This illustration shows the generalized properties of hierarchical splits. First, the projections that typically feed the split are based on a parent-child template. Hierarchical superiors get cast in the roles of ineffective parental figures: they are seen as too distant, too intrusive, or in other ways too incompetent. Conversely, caregivers are cast in the roles of children: they are seen as too immature, too soft or pliable to assume an adult-like role that demands objectivity. Second, administrators are typically denied (or deny themselves) meaningful connections to careseekers, while caregivers are denied (or deny themselves) a way to depend on administrators for support. This enables the propagation of mutually distancing projections about one another. Third, supervisors, department heads, and other middle managers avoid bringing together the other hierarchical levels; they are either absent altogether, or they have become over-identified with one level and have little connection with the other. These dynamics are consistent across caregiving organizations marked by dysfunctional hierarchical splits.

Functional splits

Caregiving organizations with functional splits are marked by similarly impermeable boundaries between functions, disciplines or professions. Organization members wall themselves off in distinct units: academic departments teaching different subjects, hospital wards dealing with different diseases or interventions, back offices dealing with financial issues or marketing, and treatment centers working with different aspects of their clients are a few examples of functional distinctions that members use to distance themselves from one another. Alternatively, members remain within boundaries defined by their particular disciplines or professions. Hospitals retain sharply defined distinctions between physicians, nurses, technicians and professional managers. Schools are marked by lines between teachers, administrators, and aides. Churches contain clergy of various training, lay leaders, and staff members. Mental health centers are marked by distinctions between psychiatrists, social workers, nurses, technicians, administrators, and support staff. Members may withdraw into their groups, defining others as outsiders against whom they need to defend their territory. Collaboration across functions, departments, and professional groups becomes difficult, as people substitute the task of marking and defending their territory in place of the primary task on which they, in connection with those they define as "other," are ostensibly working.

Roberts (1994c) describes another organization whose intergroup dynamics reveals functional splits. Staff members of a hospital medical ward were having difficulty working together across disciplinary boundaries. The occupational therapists, physiotherapists, and speech therapists were upset that when they arrived at work, their patients were still being bathed and medicated. The therapists felt sabotaged by the nurses who in turn resented being left with the heavy physical work of lifting and moving patients. The solution was reasonably simple – training therapists to help nurses with the physical work when necessary, while encouraging nurses to join in therapeutic activities on behalf of the patients. Yet the solution was difficult to get to, for it meant dismantling the social defenses that kept in play the constant blaming of one group by another. Members engaged in such blaming in order to avoid the anxiety related to their own experiences of anger and guilt triggered by the failure of patients to improve.

This example reveals some of the dynamics of functional splits. The split in the ward depends on people substituting one specialized task (e.g., bathing patients, working with their speech) for the larger primary task (i.e., improving patients' overall well-being) on which they are ostensibly joined. Members of various disciplines or departments narrow their focus to those specialized tasks; they perceive others working on their own narrowed tasks as saboteurs. The boundaries are thus drawn between, rather than around, different functional areas. Members of the different groups struggle against one another for power and resources. More broadly, they struggle for the prominence of the tasks that they deem to be primary for the unit as a whole. Collaboration is undermined.

Functional splits too are held in place because they help members avoid anxiety related to primary tasks. Members wish to locate feelings such as blame, inadequacy, sadness, and guilt elsewhere. That elsewhere lies with members of "other" groups. They use the purported differences between the groups as vehicles for splitting and projection.

Physicians believe nurses are too emotional, too subjective; nurses believe physicians are too callous, too arrogant. Mathematics teachers believe social studies teachers are not rigorous enough in their teaching of critical thinking; social studies teachers believe mathematics teachers are too distant from the lives of their students. Social workers consider psychotherapists too abstract and theoretical to be of much use to troubled clients; psychotherapists believe social workers over-identify with their clients and are unable to let them develop autonomy. The list of such mutual projections is quite long across functions, disciplines and professions.

Internal splits

Caregiving organizations may also contain intragroup splits. The drawing of boundaries that divide group members from one another marks these splits. Sub-groups or coalitions form. Members define their particular sub-group and whatever it emphasizes as primary; other sub-groups and their particular tasks are distanced and treated as "other." Individuals take on specific roles that enable the group to enact particular plays that represent the group's unspoken dilemmas (Bion 1961). Individuals are often scapegoated in the course of these enactments. Not surprisingly, this undermines the effectiveness of departments, units, and other types of work groups. As members draw away from one another and split into smaller islands they are less able to provide information and support to one another; they cannot join together to examine and interrupt ineffective ways of working on their shared tasks.

Consider the example of a staff group in a therapeutic community center for disturbed adolescents, as described by Obholzer and Roberts (1994). The weekly meetings were dominated by an ongoing conflict between two staff members. One member advocated that the staff overlook minor infractions of the rules; the second, older and more experienced, insisted on taking infractions seriously. The group considered the first member too flaky and the second too authoritarian and rigid. Other members sat back and observed the ongoing argument, frustrated or bored with it but doing little to interrupt its recurrence.

This example illustrates the dynamics that typically mark internal group splits. The group allows individual members to take up diametrically opposed positions on a key issue related to its primary task – in this case the creation of a proper relationship with clients. The group stages a play, or perhaps more to the point, a boxing match, in which a conflict central to their work is fought out by two members on behalf of all. The shared conflict is how permissive versus controlling staff members must be, a core issue in working with adolescents. The debate remains trapped within the staff group. It is located in a paralyzing conflict between two individuals and never makes its way to the surface of the organization. It becomes framed as about the conflicting individuals themselves – their personalities, their relationship – rather than as about an issue with which all members struggle.

As long as such conflicts are treated as belonging to specific individuals, other members can distance themselves from the issues implicit in those conflicts. In the illustration, staff members are able to avoid examining their experience of the tensions of working with abused children, such as that between trust and mistrust of children and parents (Obholzer & Roberts 1994). The overt conflict between two staff members, each a caricature of a position of leniency or authoritarianism, acted like a manhole cover, clamping down and keeping hidden the covert tensions that existed within each staff member in relation to their work. This is a more general process. Groups stage overt conflicts, casting about for protagonists who unconsciously agree to enable others (as well as themselves) to substitute interpersonal conflicts for more painful intrapsychic conflicts (Smith & Berg 1987). The individuals become "troublesome," for their groups and their organizations more generally, enabling the troubled system to avoid detection (Obholzer & Roberts 1994).

Identity group splits

Another type of intergroup split in caregiving organizations is that between members representing different identity groups, i.e., groups into which individuals are born, such as gender, race, ethnicity, and religion (Alderfer, 1987). Identity group splits follow a logic similar to other intergroup splits. Members draw boundaries around those who are "like them" and keep out those deemed "others." Such boundaries are drawn on the basis of enduring personal characteristics that transcend organizational groupings such as hierarchy and function. The boundaries that get drawn are, as with the other splits, inappropriate, in that they do not bring people together on behalf of their shared tasks. They are drawn to replace those tasks. Indeed, identity group splits in organizations substitute different tasks for those around which the organizations were created. They also lead to covert organizational structures that strive to replace overt structures.

This is made clearer with an illustration from Smith et al. (1989). Two women staff members in a unit of a state hospital constantly fought with and harassed one another. Their respective male supervisors, each of whom was a relatively powerful man in the organization, superficially collaborated with one another but in fact harbored resentment toward one another. They and the other men in the unit distanced themselves from the conflict, acting as if it was simply a "catfight" between the two women. The authors conducted an organizational diagnosis in which they discovered that unit members had collectively and unconsciously created a situation whereby the two women expressed conflict on behalf of all unit members. The conflict was twofold: between the powerful men, each of whom was angling for more power, and between cliques in the organization that differed in terms of the stance their members adopted in dealing with the stress of their work and the troubled state of the unit itself.

This example reveals how identity group splits are used in the service of social defenses. Unit members were collectively anxious about whether their unit would survive, given how poorly staff were working with one another and with the rest of the organization. They responded by acting as if the only way to remain protected was by maintaining the power of the men at the top of the organization. At the same time they expressed their anger by setting up two relatively low-power women to fight on behalf of the men they represented. In this fashion unit members attempted to resolve their anxiety about how to deal with the stress of their work. If one of the women "won," the stance she represented would prove correct in some way. At the same time the male leaders remained unsullied by the conflict and thus remained in protector roles. This unconscious strategy could not work, of course, since unit members could not resolve their anxiety without examining it directly. Neither woman would, or could, be allowed to "win."

Identity group splits operate on the basis of cultural images (Alderfer 1987). The hospital unit, in staging its play, appropriated a widely-held image of the powerful, protective male and the powerless, catty female. This image – like that of the angry black male, passive Asian, emotional Hispanic, and other cultural stereotypes – provided readily accessible roles that individuals could assume quite easily. It also created fault lines along which organizational members created their social defenses.

Organization/careseeker splits

Caregiving organizations may also be marked by enduring splits between organization members and those they ostensibly serve. Such splits are the clearest illustrations of how the primary task of the organization is lost: careseekers are not absorbed and digested within the system but are held at some distance. They are defined so profoundly as "others" that organization members are unable to form the attachments required to work with them as closely as they require. The social defense system in play is reasonably clear: careseekers are kept close enough to sustain the idea of their needs being met but far enough away so that the process of working with them does not trigger organization members' anxiety. This sort of split holds in place the avoidance of pain by caregivers and administrators.

Obholzer (1994), for example, describes a school for physically handicapped children in which there was a marked split between the school and the parents. The split was manifested in the form of the teachers and administrators blaming the children's difficulties on some form of parental disturbance, thereby freeing themselves of responsibility. The teachers' sense of helplessness in the face of working with profoundly handicapped children over whom they could have only limited impact and success was therefore channeled into anger and disappointment with the parents. In the course of blaming the parents they did not allow themselves the space to feel the pain associated with working with children whose health and abilities were often deteriorating. They retreated from sadness into anger. In so doing, they cut themselves off from potential allies: parents with whom they might otherwise have collaborated on behalf of the children's special needs.

A different example is found in a study by Skogstad (2000) of a medical ward specializing in cardiology. The ward was occasionally the site of sudden heart attacks and deaths. It was marked by a great deal of frenetic activity related to the constant moving of patients into, through, and out of the unit. The nurses were often quite tense, trying to monitor the patients while tending to anxious family members. In the face of such tension, the nurses and physicians developed with one another a highly sexualized atmosphere. They flirted with one another, leaning intimately close in conversation and caressing one another's hair and clothing. They excited one another. They did this in front of the patients, trying to create a culture of eroticism that pushed away the decay around them. In so doing they created an impermeable boundary between themselves as defiantly sexual, alive beings, and their ill, possibly dying, patients. In taking up their own sexuality so overtly they were defending against disturbing feelings. They reassured themselves in the face of fears of death by manically asserting life.

In each of these examples members of caregiving organizations turned away from careseekers. The teachers turned away from the parents, blaming them for their children's handicaps and deteriorations. The cardiology unit staff turned away from their patients, treating them as objects to move about rather than as humans with feelings, and turned toward one another as sources of excitement. In both cases, members are defending themselves against painful, disturbing affect: disappointment and hopelessness, distress over death. Such defenses are held in place by various projections about careseekers. In the school, the teachers framed the parents as guilty (of abuse, neglect, incompetence), the children as fatally damaged, and themselves as innocent. This enabled them to avoid examining how their work with the children might improve. In the medical ward, the staff considered their patients as bodies to be tended to, moved about and kept alive, but not as sentient beings with feelings. This framing, coupled with the intensity of their interest in one another, enabled them to avoid empathizing with, and possibly feeling the pain and anxiety of, their patients.

The paradox of resilience

Such splits within and between groups create disturbed organizational cultures. Here, culture includes both external aspects, such as work roles and practices, and the internal states of mind of individuals who take those roles and perform those practices (Trist 1990). It includes unconscious assumptions, attitudes, and beliefs about work tasks and how to perform them, that is, what Hinshelwood and Skogstad (2000: 9) describe as an "emotional atmosphere." A psychiatric ward is characterized by "touch and go" interpersonal contact between staff and patients; a school is characterized by teachers blaming parents for the children's lack of progress; a residential treatment center is characterized by staff blaming administrators for their lack of caring and resources. Each of these offers a particular type of emotional atmosphere. It becomes taken for granted, as natural and inevitable for members as the air they breathe. The fact that the atmosphere is in some fashion disturbed, that the air is not pure becomes a part of their work lives, as they go about working with one another or careseekers in ways that are patently irrational.

I have argued in this chapter that just beneath the surface of dysfunctional caregiving organizations lie various inappropriate splits between groups of members that weaken their capacities to join together and do work. These splits result from members attempting to evade anxiety. There is in play here a paradox of resilience (cf. Smith & Berg 1987). The paradox is this: it is only by moving toward anxiety that people can evade its real power to disturb them. Creating defenses against anxiety only transfigures it, locating it in different places or different forms. The anxiety remains in the organization, where it disrupts systems of caregiving. When members confront anxiety, looking squarely at where it comes from and its effects on them, they weaken its hold on them. In Part 2, I present different case studies of caregiving organizations whose members attempted to move from rather than face squarely their anxiety, and whose underlying systems of caregiving were thus disrupted in particular, all too familiar ways.

Part 2

Disturbances in caregiving organizations

Caregiving organizations struggle to respond in healthy ways to the strains of their work. They do so at the intersection of members' competing impulses. On the one hand, there is the impulse to defend against anxiety and stress, often by creating interpersonal, group and intergroup relationships that distract members from anxiety even as they are ultimately dysfunctional for them and their work. On the other hand, there is the impulse to cope with anxiety and stress by joining with others and turning together to face squarely and lessen the sources of discomfort. Patterns of behavior within caregiving organizations may often be traced to the struggle between these competing impulses; between members' desires to use one another well or badly in the course of their efforts to survive and work with careseekers.

When the struggle results in members turning away from one another in significant ways, their organizations, or units within them, become disturbed. The disturbances present themselves in various ways, according to particular organizations and their tasks, leaders, contexts, and histories. Inevitably, they drain organizational resilience. Members wall themselves off within havens they hope will keep them safe from anxiety but which cannot possibly do so. In doing this they split their organizations and undermine their collective abilities to create effective systems of caregiving.

Part 2 contains six chapters that offer particular examples of disturbances that arise in caregiving organizations and insidiously weaken their resilience. These disturbances are readily familiar. Chapter 5 presents a study of a social service agency marked by disrupted relations between social workers and administrators. Chapter 6 describes a religious-based hospital caught in widespread patterns of ineffective use of authority. Chapter 7 illustrates conflict and instability in relations between departments and units of a residential treatment center for adolescents. Chapter 8 describes a hospital's emergency care unit characterized by ineffective teamwork. Chapter 9 illustrates the corrosive effect of political behavior in the context of an urban high school. Finally, Chapter 10 presents a study of a surgical unit whose members cannot seem to change what they do and how they do it.

On the surface, these seem different organizational phenomena. Beneath the surface, however, they are much the same. Each represents a particular disturbance in members' collective capacity to stand together and work with difficult issues on behalf of careseekers. Each is the result of a collective defense against the anxiety of that work. Each also presents clues as to how dysfunctional patterns of work and interaction might be interrupted and members helped to create more resilient ways to working together. These clues are interpreted and worked with more closely in Part 3.

Chapter 5

Caregivers and casualties

Caregivers are notoriously susceptible to burnout. Their work demands empathic relationships and often a great deal of emotional involvement. They risk being emotionally drained, giving of themselves until they have nothing more to give. This is known as job burnout, in which people are physically or emotionally exhausted, negative about themselves and their jobs, and increasingly less concerned about their clients (Pines & Maslach 1978). They become depersonalized and emotionally withdrawn. Burnout research focuses on the various causes and manifestations of such withdrawals and the resulting implications for work effectiveness, morale, and turnover (Maslach 1982).

The literature on job burnout advocates various interventions to halt the depersonalization of caregivers. One type of intervention focuses on shoring up their personal defenses against burnout with, for example, time outs at work, professional skill development, and learning appropriately detached stances (Cherniss 1980). These mechanisms enable caregivers to remove themselves emotionally when they are in danger of being emptied. Another type of intervention focuses on peer support groups inside and outside the workplace (Maslach 1982) and supervision that offers feedback, technical assistance, and support (Pines & Aronson 1988). These interventions allow caregivers to be, for a time, careseekers and have others personally attend to them in the service of their growth and healing. These strategies are particularly effective when they enable caregivers to experience themselves as cared for at work, which replenishes their "supplies" of emotional caring. Seen thus, the caregiving organization itself – through the structures of peer group and supervisory meetings – can enable its caregivers to be appropriately ministered to. If these structures are absent, the chances of burnout are increased.

This suggests the more general proposition noted earlier. Caregivers may be filled with or emptied of emotional resources in the course of their interactions with other organization members, which shape their abilities to perform their roles effectively. This makes explicit what is implicit in job burnout literature: the extent to which caregivers are held within their own organizations affects their abilities to hold others similarly. This is the organizational analogue to Gaylin's (1976: 63) statement "To be cared for is essential for the capacity to be caring." It reflects Lyth's (1988) ideas about caregiving organizations as therapeutic milieu, in which the quality of patient or client care depends on the extent to which an institution as a whole becomes therapeutic and its members model caregiving behaviors toward one another. Lyth (1988: 253) found that staff members of children's institutions were most effective at their tasks when they "experience the same concern and support for their stresses as they are expected to provide for children and their families," when they were "given opportunities for mature functioning," and when they were "contained in a system of meaningful attachments."

Relational systems

Resilient caregiving organizations are marked by functional *relational systems*, in which there is the potential for each and every member to be contained in a meaningful attachment. Meaningful attachments are those that resemble, between adults, the type of secure attachments described in Chapter 1 between parents and children. Organization members are able to take risks, challenge themselves, and enter emotionally difficult territory, secure in the knowledge that others will come to their aid should the need arise. In parent-child relationships, of course, this is relatively unambiguous; authority lies in the hands of the parent, on whom the child is generally dependent, until they gradually negotiate different relationships. In adult work relationships the process is more ambiguous, and coexists within a constellation of competing relationships (i.e., managing, reporting, coaching, supervising, and peer). Nevertheless, the opportunity exists for all members to have relationship lifelines onto which they can grab and let themselves be pulled into shore by others not as caught up in anxiety-arousing situations.

There are also dysfunctional relational systems. In these, all members do not have access to a meaningful, secure attachment. They may be involved in insecure attachments or in none at all. Insecure attachments are those in which secure base relations have been disrupted or prevented from occurring (Bowlby 1980). This tends to happen in one or both of two ways (Kahn 1998). People may be *abandoned* by others who withdraw from, ignore, are insensitive to or in other ways turn away from their experiences and expressed needs. Or people may be *intruded* on by others, who interrupt, project onto, take over, substitute for or in other ways obliterate their experiences and expressed needs. When people intrude upon others they silence them: they push away their experiences and act as if others' internal lives do not exist or do not matter. Both processes leave individuals isolated from others. They are left unseen, unknown, metaphorically dropped rather than held.

The ongoing abandonment of or intrusion on some group or sub-set of an organization marks dysfunctional relational systems. Members of a group, department, functional area, or identity group are left without relationships in which they can safely voice anxiety and make meaning of events that seem confusing, crazy, or in other ways upsetting. Their lack of attachments is related not to their own particular inclinations, abilities, or situations but to a larger pattern woven into their organizations. The pattern holds that, for some segment of the organization, attachment relationships are prevented or disrupted. Groups or sub-groups are left unprotected and vulnerable. While the system might be functional for some members, the relational system as a whole is dysfunctional: it sacrifices some of its members, leaving them as casualties.

In this chapter I examine how and why meaningful attachments between caregivers – teachers, therapists, social workers, nurses, physicians, clergy – and others within their organizations are disrupted. I show how easily caregivers can become casualties. In the covert war against the anxiety of working with careseekers, primary caregivers are on the front lines. In dysfunctional organizations they are left there, isolated, without the support necessary to maintain their effectiveness. They are not held closely enough within a system of caregiving. This has implications for their work, their relations with those they serve, and for their organizations more generally.

Project Home

Project Home was a social service agency that provided homeless children (aged 8–17) with responsible adult volunteers as role models (for more detail, see Kahn 1993, 1995, 1998). Agency members raised funds from private, public, and charitable sources, located and screened potential youths and adults, formed and supervised approximately 350 matches, worked with government agencies to deal with troubled youths, and conducted programs to train, engage, and celebrate volunteers. A board of directors (approximately 40 members) served as a network of fundraisers, and its various committees were charged with overseeing strategy, investments, and staff issues. For all practical purposes, however, the agency's director oversaw daily operations and long-term strategic decisions. The agency staff included, besides the director, the fundraiser (liaison to corporate and foundation contacts), office manager, social worker supervisor, and the social workers as the primary caregivers of the matches made between volunteers and youths. Agency members worked from a central office, although some social workers were assigned to branch offices scattered about the region.

At the time of the study the agency was undergoing a difficult period financially, given a local and national recession that affected charitable contributions, and was involved in an endowment campaign to raise capital to supplement the annual operating budget. Staff turnover was high. During my contact with the agency, four of six social workers, their supervisor, and the secretary left and were replaced (after some delay), and the assistant fundraiser left and was not replaced. A senior social worker calculated that 14 social workers (of a staff of 7) had left in the preceding 28-month period. The turnover undermined consistent relationships with clients, many of whom slipped through the cracks left by revolving personnel. One social worker noted, "A lot of us get files that have been passed around and around." Another told of calling a volunteer who reported that his charge had been in the youth services lock-up for two years, which no one at the agency had known or recorded.

Over the course of a year I analyzed Project Home's *relational system*: the patterns of caregiving that occurred among agency members (see Kahn 1993). The relational system was marked by two predominant patterns. First, no caregiving flowed from the administrative (director, fundraiser, office manager) to the caregiving (supervisor, social workers) branches of the agency. The only attachment between the two branches was a relatively weak one between the director and the supervisor, with the latter occasionally reaching out to the former during administrative meetings. Second, the social workers provided caregiving to their clients and to their supervisor but were themselves bereft of caregiving, except for that which they informally gave to one another. Such self-replenishment, while useful, had its limits. The social workers were a closed sub-system, with little caregiving from others, and they often exhausted their collective resources with one another. In the short term, social workers were generally able to usefully serve their clients. Their energies were slowly drained, however, in spite of their efforts otherwise. In the long term they became emotionally overdrawn, and at some point disengaged – withdrew, became cynical, or left altogether – in the face of burnout.

The social workers were left isolated in the context of their relationships with the director, supervisor, and administrators. This is illustrated in the following sections, using data originally reported elsewhere (Kahn 1993).

Director-social workers relationship

The relationship between the director and social workers was marked by mutual animosity and withdrawal of support. The director perceived the social workers as largely "irresponsible," unwilling to "take ownership of their work and their mistakes." He also perceived the social workers as "out to get [him], always making [him] the bad guy." The social workers perceived the director as "cold" and "manipulative," "caring more about numbers than about the kids or [social workers]," and unwilling to allow them to meaning-fully participate in relevant decisions. The relationship remained caught in the web of these mutual perceptions, to the point that agency members were largely unable to see or believe evidence that contradicted their images of the other party. They became locked within self-fulfilling prophecies, behaving in ways that elicited from others exactly the behaviors that confirmed their beliefs about others as well as those about themselves.

An illustration of this pattern occurred when the executive director called and led an impromptu supervision meeting for the social workers. His stated agenda was to find out how new matches between the youths and volunteers were progressing. Much of the meeting, however, involved the executive director talking about projects he envisioned for the agency's future. The meeting was a study in the mutual withholding of care. The executive director did not inquire about, listen to or empathize with the social workers' experiences of feeling understaffed, overwhelmed, and needing support. Nor did he encourage them, offer positive feedback, show respect for their efforts, or provide support in the form of minimal resources or compassion. There was a similar lack of caregiving going from social workers toward the executive director. They did not inquire about, listen to, or empathize with his having to steer the agency through a difficult economic period nor show positive encouragement and respect for his efforts. They too offered no support or compassion. The meeting included the following interchange.

Director: And the board and [board president] are very supportive of us continuing to raise money to fund these new programs. [*Extended silence*] Anything else before we leave?

Social worker 1:   How are we going to have enough social workers to staff these new programs? We've barely enough people and time to do what we're doing now.

Director: We're projecting that the economy will allow us to hire more people next year.

Social worker 2:   Next year? I thought we were going to be hiring two new full-time people this year.

Director: We're not hiring new staff this year. We have a policy here in the agency to never hire staff that we might have to let go because of the economy. We've never had to cut back in the years I've been here. It's just too tricky now with the economy.

Social worker 3:   But you told us that we would be able to hire more people and get some help. Two people just left in the last two months.

Social worker 1:   Let me get this straight. We won't be hiring any more full-time social workers?

Director: Not right now.

Social worker 3:   Isn't that why we didn't get raises this year? So we can use the money to fund new staff? That's what you said before.

Social worker 4:   Why weren't we told this before?

Social worker 1:   What about [the social worker supervisor]? When will she be coming back?

Director:	As you know, we've just hired a replacement. She will be joining us next month.
Social worker 1:	The memo you sent us didn't indicate that she [the new supervisor] was a temporary replacement and how she and [the former supervisor] would work together.
Director:	[The former supervisor] will not be coming back in her present capacity. [The new supervisor] will be the full-time social worker supervisor. I had already told this group that.
Social worker 4:	What?
Social worker 3:	When? No one told us anything.
Director:	I had communicated that before.
Social worker 2:	Then why don't any of us here know? Did we all simply repress that information?
Director:	Yes. You're forgetting what I've said before.
Social worker 1 [laughs]:	I don't think so. You never told us that she [the former supervisor] wasn't coming back.

This interchange was characterized by mutual frustration, bitterness, and withholding. The participants talked at different levels of abstraction. The executive director spoke abstractly and unemotionally ("We're projecting that the economy ...") while the social workers spoke in terms of concrete immediacy ("We've barely enough people and time to do what we're doing now"), and particular emotions (e.g., frustration, outrage). The two parties did not connect with one another; rather than pause to carefully inquire into one another's experiences, they escalated until the interaction resembled a team of prosecutors barraging a witness with questions. Like sophisticated trial lawyers, the social workers simultaneously sought to extract information while showing disbelief in the witness and trying to trip him up in inconsistencies. The executive director assumed the role of hostile witness, retreating to a defensive position. Ultimately he retreated to the position of the authority figure whose word must be accepted on its own terms, leaving the social workers in the role of frustrated, angry subordinates.

The social workers reacted to the director in various ways. Some confronted him, trying to have him understand and respond to their concerns and experiences. This was invariably unsuccessful. Over time they became angry ("He's shutting people down, shutting me down, and it's infuriating") and sad ("It makes me feel very demoralized"). They retreated emotionally from interactions involving the director. One social worker noted about a meeting, for example, "I thought that ultimately it doesn't matter what any of us have to say. It made me just want to give up." Most social workers at some point withdrew in their relations with the director; as one social worker noted, "Now I just pay no attention, go about my business, try not to get too involved with him." Such withdrawals (which became permanent as social workers quit the agency) reflected their response to a relationship with their director in which support and caregiving were unforthcoming. The social workers looked elsewhere for support, most notably, to their supervisor.

Supervisor-social workers relationship

The supervisor and the social workers liked and valued one another while abdicating their roles of supervisor and supervisee. This abdication assumed a variety of forms, ranging from the supervisor not representing the social workers' interests to the administrators, to the social workers taking care of their supervisor without reciprocation. The following excerpt from a group supervision meeting, whose agenda included a discussion of the social workers' anxieties and concerns, illustrates the relationship between the supervisor and the social worker group.

Supervisor: I don't have any particular structure so we can talk about what you want.

Social worker 1:   What are we supposed to be talking about?

Social worker 2:   We're here to talk about concerns, feelings, issues about the agency.

Supervisor: From my angle things haven't gone right because of time. We've had so many new people starting at the same time, and I've been so tired. It takes time to get things back to normal. I'm not moving at a fast pace.

Social worker 1:   How are you feeling?

Supervisor: Okay, not great. Tired. Look, we need to figure out what to do, how to have it better, easier. It's not going to happen overnight.

Social worker 3:   Things get changed back and forth all the time around here. It's impossible to have a conversation with [director]. It doesn't go anywhere, and you're always on the losing end.

Supervisor: I've been so swamped. We just need to get the systems working right, how we communicate with each other about events. You're all working so hard and so well.

Social worker 2:   It's more than that. There's just too much inconsistency around here. We never know what's going to happen from day to day.

Social worker 4:   We don't have any idea of what's going to happen when you go on your maternity leave.

Supervisor: I don't think there's a plan yet. I haven't heard of one.

Social worker 4:   That's completely unacceptable.

Social worker 1:   That's crazy.

Social worker 5:   I just want to go into my office and close the door.

Social worker 2:   I feel like I want to have a buddy, like in the old buddy
                      system.
Social worker 3:   It's called peer supervision when you get to be an adult.

This passage illustrates the supervisor's habitual ways of interacting
with the social workers. She sat with them and listened to them. She was
appreciative of their work ("You're all working so hard and so well"). Yet her
positive emotion was not often grounded in empathic understanding. (As one
social worker noted, the supervisor was "Very positive, very validating,
although you get a sense she doesn't quite know what you're doing or what
you're skills are"). The supervisor did not fully take in and digest the social
workers' experiences. She limited her intake by focusing on administrative
rather than emotional issues ("We just need to get the systems working
right"), switching away from reviewing their experiences ("It's impossible")
to her own ("I've been so swamped"), and rationalizing or simplifying rather
than digging for difficult experiences. The supervisor abandoned the social
workers by limiting her support of them, in terms of training and feedback.
She also abandoned them not only by not attending to them more fully but by
not helping them create a sense of consistency ("We never know what's going
to happen from day to day"), providing information ("I don't think there's a
plan yet"), and offering protection ("You're always on the losing end"). The
supervisor exhibited what one social worker referred to as "controlled,
limited caring" that undermined her ability to support, advocate for and be a
secure base for the social workers.

The social workers reacted in particular ways. They became self-sufficient,
withdrawing from expressing their needs to their supervisor ("I just want to
go into my office and close the door"). As one noted, "We care for ourselves
here." They simplified the problems they brought to their supervisor until
supervision became, as one described, "just like reporting." A social worker
noted, "I don't bring to her lots of conflicts. I always bring my suggested
resolutions and usually it's what she thinks. I leave the harder ones out." The
social workers found themselves offering care to their supervisor, giving her
support – in effect, performing a sort of parent-child role inversion described
by family systems theorists (Bowlby 1988; Miller 1981). They colluded with
the supervisor's abdication of her role as their anchor, the person to whom
they could legitimately turn for support, protection, and nurturing at
appropriate moments. They implied their need for help and support without
explicitly turning to her as a provider – as if they already knew her limits in
that regard and wished to spare themselves disappointment and rejection.

Administrators-social workers relationship

The relationship between the lower-level administrators (i.e., fundraiser,
office manager, assistant fundraiser, secretary) and the social workers was

marked by a gulf in which members of each group felt disrespected by, unheard by and disconnected from members of the other group. The gulf was shaped by the perceptions that members of each group held. The administrators perceived the social workers as naive, demanding, oblivious to the financial aspects of their agency, and irresponsible. They perceived themselves as responsible, fiscally aware and struggling to keep the agency afloat, and the social workers as demanding and needy, childishly unaware of the fundamental issues of agency survival. For their part, the social workers perceived the administrators as caring more about numbers – grants secured, funds spent, clients served – than about the youths the agency sought to serve. The social workers perceived themselves as being on the front lines of a struggle with difficult issues (e.g., child abuse, split families), and having their time and energy wasted by administrators who cared more about paperwork than the clients or the social workers themselves. These various perceptions led administrators and social workers alike to feel neither supported nor valued by the other.

Interactions between the social workers and administrators were shaped by these mutual perceptions. The following excerpt from a staff meeting, in which the social workers are seeking support and help, illustrates key dimensions of their relationship.

Social worker 1:   We [social workers] met and talked about our concerns about communication here. We wanted to see what the others thought.

Social worker 2:   I mean, we're wondering if others in the agency are having thoughts about it.

Office manager: Wasn't it the social workers' meeting that brought all this stuff up?

Social worker 1:   It's not just us that have these feelings and concerns.

Fundraiser: We're small but we're growing and we need to address that but not in a crisis fashion. As adults. We need to just sit down, as adults, and think about what we can do to make this a better agency. There is a positive basis that has already been built up. You need to approach it like that.

Social worker 3:   We are talking about this as adults. We're not just bringing these concerns like kids, here, fix this. We want to see if others in the agency feel these things.

Office manager: I feel hassled a lot. Like I'm not getting a lot of support and tolerance from others. The phone rings, no one gets it. I'm eating lunch, and you [social workers] barge in on me. I also have a lot of my own stuff to do.

Social worker 2:   I get blown off a lot by the staff here too, like when I'm trying to keep up with the paperwork and need help.

Secretary: People are late with their documentation [case write-ups]. I can't keep up with that, can't hound you or clean up after you. Sometimes I can't even find you.

Social worker 1:   I'm sorry. I'm guilty there. But I can't see doing all that paperwork when I'm running around trying to get kids matched up and supervised. That doesn't seem to be the priority here.

Fundraiser: It's a priority. Of course. But we have to look at the bigger picture. Which we do, so you don't have to.

This passage shows the social workers raising issues and concerns that were only partially acknowledged by the administrators as related to them. The social workers were, in effect, calling out for help, seeking administrators' assistance in understanding the agency's dysfunctional patterns of communication. They were met with rebuffs ("Wasn't it the social workers . . .?"), a desire for suppression ("There is a positive basis") and various statements emphasizing adult/child projections ("As adults", "Clean up after you"). The administrators cast off rather than reached out to the social workers. The social workers responded in kind. They withheld information from the administrators (case documents), intruded upon the office manager ("You barge in on me"), disrupted the secretary's schedule ("I can't keep up with that") and withdrew from interactions altogether ("Sometimes I can't even find you").

Moments of caregiving did occur between administrators and social workers during one-on-one interactions. These occurred in the context of relationships developed over a relatively long period of time. For example, the most senior social worker and the fundraiser were increasingly able to support one another in small, fleeting ways (e.g., inquiring about events, borrowing an office or phone, donating clothing) after they were colleagues for three years. Similarly, the office manager and another social worker developed a personal connection, in which they too had caring moments (e.g., bringing coffee to one another, debriefing agency events and situations). Yet, all told, these interactions did not develop the larger capacity of the administrators and social workers to connect across the sub-group boundary. Such support remained at the periphery rather than at the core of the agency.

Implications for social workers

The social workers sought to create meaningful attachments among themselves. They felt that they had little choice but to turn to one another for caregiving. In so doing they cut themselves off from other parts of the organization that failed to provide adequate caregiving, becoming caregivers for themselves as well as their clients.

This pattern is illustrated by a monthly group supervision meeting the social workers led for themselves. The supervisor led these regularly scheduled meetings but when she was unavailable the social workers facilitated their own meeting rather than have the executive director lead the meeting or postpone it altogether. The meeting contained the following interchanges.

Social worker 1 (facilitator): What else?

Social worker 2: It's been hard to get hold of the volunteers; they don't seem to get their messages or return my calls a lot of the time. It's frustrating.

Social worker 3: I know what you mean. It is frustrating. It sometimes helps to leave messages saying exactly when they can call you, so they don't think they have to waste their time trying.

Social worker 1: When you reach them, how do you find the conversations?

Social worker 4: Sometimes people don't offer much. I'm afraid to put words in their mouths. I don't want to feed them when we talk; I want them to talk on their own.

Social worker 2: I know, it can get like pulling teeth. Sometimes it's important just to stay on the phone with them sometimes, just to build the relationship. After a time, it gets easier.

Social worker 3: I think that's right. It lets them know that they have some place to go to when they need to.

Social worker 1: I was thinking that it would be useful to flag some issues and how to deal with them. I was thinking about a mother who called me and was beside herself because the volunteer was letting her child sit on his lap and drive the car. What would you do with that?

Social worker 5: The mother is the one who has to feel okay about her child's match. I would try to affirm and legitimate her perspective and hear what's going on for her.

Social worker 2: I agree. You would have to build rapport with her if she is going to work with you to support the match.

Social worker 3 [rising to close the conference room door]: There is so much potential for mothers to sabotage the matches. You have to support her and establish a connection with her, so if she's overly worried you can reason with her later.

Social worker 1: That was exactly my experience with this case.

Social worker 6: Can I ask about a case I have? It involves a sexually abused child who is not talking about it with his volunteer.

Social worker 1: Let's help. What's going on?

Social worker 6: The boy just won't open up and the volunteer is concerned.

Social worker 5: It may be that when the kid is with the volunteer he

	doesn't want to be a victim or a witness, he just wants to be a kid.
Social worker 1:	And what's probably important here is to get the volunteer himself to talk about his own feelings about the situation. Perhaps the way to help the boy is to make sure that the volunteer isn't pressing him to talk because of his own needs, and that he can be available to the boy when the time comes.
Social worker 3:	Which means that you have to be available to the volunteer in the same way, not just pressuring him to talk but letting him know that he's in a difficult situation and he may be having his own reactions to it. And you're there if he needs to talk about it.
Social worker 4:	Yeah. Sometimes it's just about us helping the volunteers realize that their feelings are important in these situations too.
Social worker 6:	That all makes sense. Thanks. I'll work on it with him.
Social worker 1:	We need to wrap this up. Anything else?
Social worker 2:	I'd like to thank you for doing an outstanding job of running the meeting. (*Others applaud*).

In this meeting the social workers set up boundaries (i.e., requesting that the executive director be absent, closing the door), literally and figuratively creating the space in which to care for themselves. Within that space they shared emotions and experiences. They explored issues and emotions. The facilitator posed questions ("What would you do with that?"), joined with others ("That was exactly my experience with this case"), and suggested rather than imposed direction ("Perhaps the way to help the boy is to . . ."). The other social workers followed suit. Together, they worked on the task of caring for youths and volunteers and created a care structure for themselves. The structure dissolved as the social workers re-entered the organization looking for direction, information, and resources. Even there they looked more to one another than to their nominal superiors. They were caught in a double bind. If they did not become self-contained they were bereft of caregiving; when they did become self-contained they distanced themselves further from others, and were distanced by them in return.

The social workers were, by and large, left relatively isolated in the agency. As one social worker noted:

It's like its all individual here. No one is looking at the system or the whole or the community. Everyone is out for themselves. That's in some sense how I'm functioning now; I have to take care of myself. There's no system to give to or get back from. There's no circle to join, nothing that

I can be part of, there's no whole. I do a lot of reality checks, to make sure that I'm not crazy.

The isolation – the "nothing [to] be part of" – held implications for the social workers' work, burnout, and turnover. It was difficult for them to be emotionally present when they were tending to clients *and* coping with the lack of support in their own agency. Social workers conducting constant "reality checks" with one another and devising effective strategies to deal with agency relationships were less present for their clients. Time spent huddling about how to deal with the latest perceived insult, administrative policy, or agency dynamic was time not spent with clients. Emotional energies expended in dealing with their isolation took them away from working with clients' more painful emotions. They withdrew from such difficult emotional work ("After a while I find myself not making difficult calls I should be making. I'll call people whose matches I know are going well"). They were late completing necessary documentation, unwilling to get involved in agency-wide activities and slow to develop solutions to lingering problems. They traced such withdrawal to their treatment in the agency. One noted, "I know that if I were receiving more I would be better here. There's a lot of potential that I have that isn't being nurtured here and everyone suffers."

(Dys)functions served

The overall system of relationships among Project Home members was markedly inefficient, even irrational, given the agency's task of providing ongoing care for youth-adult relationships. That task required ongoing, secure attachments between social workers and their clients, who were already feeling skittish in relation to loss and abandonment. The turnover of social workers clearly disrupted client relationships. So why did this system of organizational caregiving exist? The story that agency members told revolved around the notion of understaffing. Since social workers were not immediately replaced after they left, those who were left had to manage more cases. They were overworking. They had little time and emotional energy to expend in caregiving with one another. The understaffing created a self-perpetuating cycle in the agency. Newly-hired social workers were overwhelmed with work, had difficulty forming attachments with veteran administrators, burned out and left, and were replaced with others, *ad infinitum*.

While this story had currency within the agency it was also a cover for a more complicated dynamic. The agency divided, in essence, into two staffs, one consisting of long-term administrators and the other of short-term, "journeymen" social workers who flowed in and out without being taken into the core of the agency. This set-up ensured a lack of secure attachments between the two sub-systems and led to the unintended isolation and emotional abandonment of the social workers. This dynamic served particular functions. As noted previously, patterns of behavior within and between groups which remain in place, even as they are seemingly destructive to their given tasks, serve functions. Irrational patterns serve irrational functions, or rather, dysfunctions. Such was the case for the set of relationships between the groups of Project Home.

Project Home's set of relationships served two primary functions. First, isolating the social workers located painful emotions in them rather than in other members. As agency members with the most direct, sustained, and frequent contact with the clients, the social workers most keenly experienced the anxiety related to working with homeless, often destitute and abandoned, needy and dependent youths. They experienced painful feelings: rage at parents who left their children, sorrow for the youths and parents left behind, fear about matching youths with potentially abusive volunteers, fear of being overwhelmed by the youths' neediness, and hopelessness about the enormity of homeless children needing help. They were left stuck with those painful emotions and anxieties. The administrators suffered as well, in a different fashion. They were left complaining about not feeling emotionally connected to the homeless youths they wished to help. This disconnection was the price they paid for remaining relatively detached from the social workers' experiences.

This first function was, of course, defensive. Individuals defend themselves against anxiety by absenting or sacrificing parts of themselves, detaching emotional "limbs" that would otherwise bring them in contact with troubling emotions and anxiety (Freud 1936). The agency operated in much the same way, at a different level. The social workers' splitting off from the rest of the organization was an involuntary sacrifice that kept agency administrators – as the ongoing core of the agency, given social worker turnover – protected from seemingly debilitating anxiety, which they unconsciously feared would destroy the agency if it was experienced too directly. The social workers, as primary caregivers, waded out into a river of painful emotions to help rescue homeless youths, and the other parts of the agency, instead of pulling taut on the lifeline connecting and anchoring the social workers to the organization, unconsciously dropped the rope and abandoned the social workers to the force of the waves so as not be pulled in themselves. The social workers lacked the status and political power in the agency to halt the process. Their turnover ensured that the process continued. The anxiety itself did not dissipate but instead was deflected into the relationships between the social workers and the director, supervisor, and administrators.

The second function served by Project Home's relational system was to provide a nuanced set of data about their clients' experiences. The social workers empathized with their clients, to the point that they had some sense of what they felt – loss, abandonment, anger, sadness. They experienced these feelings in the natural course of developing relationships with the youths and families. They imported those feelings into the agency and the feelings drove the covert play that agency members staged. They interacted with one another in ways that paralleled families in which the father (as head of the household) was absent and the children felt homeless. Agency members acted toward one another "as if" they were such a family. The director was the *absent father*: a distant, emotionally unavailable, uncaring male head of household who focused on the financial (i.e., fundraising) rather than the emotional needs of his family. The supervisor was the *overwhelmed mother*: exhausted, abandoned by the father to provide, weakly, the nurturing (i.e., clinical supervision) to the children. The social workers were the needy, isolated, and abandoned *children*: deprived of adequate emotional support from the absent father and over-whelmed mother, disempowered by their lack of connections with the agency and their lack of voice in decision-making processes.

That these roles so closely mirrored those of the families the agency served suggested a *parallel process*, in which the emotions and behaviors of one system are paralleled in another (Alderfer 1987). Agency members unconsciously recreated the dynamics of the families with which they worked. The social workers working closely with homeless children took their anger at the fathers who in many cases had abandoned their families, and projected it onto the director, a likely candidate given his position of author-ity and his seeming absence from agency members. He stood in for the absent fathers, toward whom anger could not be directly expressed. The social work-ers expressed anger at the director both actively (e.g., blaming him for work-loads) and passively (e.g., not completing necessary documentation). They cast their supervisor as the stand-in for the overwhelmed, abandoned mothers. They perceived her as fragile, unable to handle the demands of her workload and pregnancy. They withheld feedback and kept her out of decision-making loops, noting that it was in her best interests. The supervisor colluded with the projections about her weakness and ineffectiveness by tell-ing social workers that the director was the source of their problems. The social workers cast themselves in the role of homeless youths, deprived of adequate emotional support from the absent father and overwhelmed mother. Disempowered by their lack of connections with the agency and their lack of voice in decision-making processes, they were, organizationally, as "homeless" as the clients they served.

Agency members collectively staged this play for their own benefit. Like members of many caregiving organizations, they were unconsciously import-ing the emotions, situations, and experiences of those they served, the better to recreate and understand them. This was a communication process, using the projective identification mechanism described in Chapter 2. This function is informative rather than defensive. Project Home members had the opportunity to examine within the laboratory of their own agency the experi-ences of their clients. In resilient organizations administrators and other members join with caregivers to interpret that information. This did not occur at Project Home. Its members were unable to understand that they were collectively, unconsciously, enacting a covert play. Instead they simply continued the play. To maintain its lengthy run they reinforced sharp, inappropriate divisions between the administrators and social workers. They were unable to step back and reflect on the play they enacted, to examine it as a re-presentation of client dynamics from which they could learn a great deal about how to better perform their work.

Reclaiming the casualties

This example illustrates a type of systemic disruption that splits off primary caregivers from the rest of the organization. On the surface, caregivers burn out, exhausted by the intensity and strain of their work. Beneath the surface, caregivers are often casualties in their organizations' war against the anxiety of working with clients, patients, students, and other careseekers. They may be more or less wounded in their work, dealing with painful situations. But in dysfunctional caregiving systems like Project Home it is not those wounds that destroy caregivers, it is being left behind by their organizations. Frost (2003) offers a compelling analysis of pain in organizations – its inevitability, its manifestations – and suggests that it becomes toxic to members when others respond to it without compassion. At Project Home, the social workers were dropped rather than held. Wading into the oceans of careseekers, they turned and saw others drop the lifelines and walk away toward the safety of the dunes. They were left there as surely as if they were front-line troops left wounded in enemy territory, the helicopters whirring away, leaving them for dead.

Often enough, caregivers isolated within their organizations regroup to develop their own support systems. Teachers coalesce in teacher lounges, sharing stories and venting emotions. Social workers, staff therapists and counselors, and healthcare workers provide peer supervision and support. Clergy attend conferences at which they might participate in workshops with one another. These activities are important. They are also limited in their long-term effectiveness. Unless paired with supportive relationships with members from other parts of the organization, caregivers tend to create self-sealing, closed systems that exacerbate rather than alleviate stress. They need secure attachments to others who are less caught up in the emotional connection to careseekers. They need, in short, to be held and contained by others that parallel how they are with careseekers. When teachers, social workers, therapists, and healthcare workers complain that they are overwhelmed and under-appreciated by their organizations they are voicing their experiences of not being taken in, attended to and cared for in ways necessary to enable them to continue their work.

When caregivers are reclaimed, no longer the casualties of social defenses, inappropriate boundaries are dismantled. The caregivers are gathered up, held onto by other caregiving organization members. They are no longer unconsciously perceived as "acceptable losses" that protect the ongoing core of the organization at the expense of expendable others. They are brought in, as part of the organization. Caregivers and administrators maintain meaningful connections.

In practice, this occurs when members look together at their patterns of behavior and struggle to understand how and why they are locked into certain perceptions and practices. This sort of understanding leads to the interruption of dysfunctional behavior. People have to be led to and through this process. Leaders such as Project Home's executive director may decide to push for change, spurred by increasingly unacceptable losses in effectiveness or personnel. Or members, such as the social workers, may agitate up through the ranks, beginning with their supervisor and sympathetic administrators, until the executive director, shamed or challenged, has little choice but to begin some sort of change process. The process may involve outside consultation, which would help leaders and members interrupt their taken-for-granted assumptions and perceptions about one another that blocked their shared understanding of the particular stress and anxiety under which they had all been operating.

Interrupting the patterns of a system like that of Project Home will require, at the least, three phases. First, members and leaders need to explore the possibility that the perceptions they have of one another and their behaviors toward one another are shaped by careseekers' emotions that stream into and lie just beneath the surface of the organization. They must play with this idea, acting as if it might be true, using it as a lens through which to view their relations and perceptions. They will need help to do this, by consultants who help them think about the roles into which they cast one another – absent father, overwhelmed mother, abandoned children – and how those roles parallel their clients. When they understand, and then understand again, their unconscious mirroring of their clients, they may then choose to learn from that mirroring. They can learn of their clients' experiences, their hopes and fears, their particular stress and anxiety – and use that information to better empathize with and care for them.

Second, members and leaders need to speak the truth of their emotional experiences to one another – their sense of failure, of guilt and shame, anger and resentment; their twin desires to save and cast off clients; their longing for and distrust of connections within the agency. It is against these emotional experiences that Project Home members defend, by creating dysfunctional relations that render all of them, in one fashion or another, casualties, with the social workers the most observably harmed. To the extent that members are able to make transparent those experiences to one another, and work to support rather than castigate one another, they may have less need to use one another in harmful ways. The work here is for Project Home members to let go of their desires to blame particular individuals, to construct narratives that hold them, rather than the nature of their work and clients, at the center of their explanations for their distress. They will need help with this, given that they remain locked within narratives that have over time calcified into standard, taken-for-granted beliefs about one another. They will also need to give feedback to one another that points out the particular roles that they play. It is only through such feedback that awareness may develop, and with it, the potential for insight and change.

Finally, members and leaders will need ongoing forums in which to regularly reflect upon and speak of their experiences in the agency. Such forums – regular full staff meetings, group supervisions, and administrative meetings – allow people to routinely understand the stress that presses down upon each person in the agency. These forums must be led in particular ways. A consultant can set the tone in the first few meetings, creating ground rules that allow for relatively safe conversations. Gradually, this can give way to members assuming the responsibility for facilitating meetings that have as their aim not simply complaint but understanding and insight. Organizations such as Project Home must develop the capacity for members to meet regularly to reflect upon their work experiences, to examine the particular anxieties that attend their work, and their impulses to defend against them in their relations with one another. Without such forums, built into both organizational structures and, given time, cultures, people are doomed to act out against rather than alleviate their underlying anxieties. This does damage to individuals, careseekers, and the organizations themselves.

Every caregiving organization faces a crucial choice point in relation to how its caregivers are brought into or held away from its core. The choice is about how to authorize caregivers. In Project Home, the social workers were unable to halt their own isolation because they lacked the power to do so. This is a hallmark of dysfunctional relational systems. Caregivers most directly provide the services that define and give existence to their organizations but are the least powerful and often the least valued by those who wield authority. Social workers, nurses, teachers, residential care workers, and childcare workers often have little authority in their organizations, and to the extent that they do, it is often because they belong to unions that advance their cause (while maintaining adversarial relations within the organization). They lack the authority to dismantle the inappropriate boundaries that wall them off from others in their organizations. The leadership task, as described in Part 3, involves holding caregivers close enough to enable them to influence their organizations. It involves keeping them safely inside.

Chapter 6

Authority at work

Caregiving organizations, like other types of organization, are marked by their members' constant struggles to use authority in appropriate ways. Organizational authority refers to the right to do work within the boundaries of organizational roles (Gould 1993), or more concretely, to make decisions which are binding on others (Obholzer 1994). Formal authority is derived from organizational roles and is exercised on behalf of organizations. Used appropriately, such authority is rooted in and serves primary tasks. Physicians direct nurses and technicians to medicate patients in certain ways, school principals create guidelines for new programs they expect teachers to follow, clergy create outlines for religious services that require certain administrative duties to be carried out by staff members, residential treatment coordinators develop systems for integration that require childcare workers to follow certain protocols, and social service agency directors expect supervisors to translate new state policies into new social worker practices. In each case, individuals located in certain work roles and hierarchical positions delegate activities to individuals located in other roles and positions.

Organizational hierarchies require such delegation. It is the means by which leaders "lend" authority to others, enabling them to participate in the leadership process (Hirschhorn 1997). Those individuals, in turn, restrict their own autonomy on behalf of organizational needs. They trade some of their personal authority – their rights to authentically express and enact themselves as they see fit (Gould 1993) – for a system of organizational authority, in which they delegate and are delegated to in order to work with others on shared organizational tasks.

This process presumes rationality. It presupposes that people willingly subordinate parts of themselves to organizational hierarchies that appropriately direct and focus their energies. It also presupposes that the processes by which hierarchies function are transparently dictated by the requirements of organizational tasks and the coordination mechanisms they require. Rationally, leaders are supported by followers who take up their own personal and organizational authority to protect parts of their organizations (Hirschhorn 1997). Leaders and followers are willingly dependent on one another. Their mutual trust is ideally rewarded by a trustworthy, functioning hierarchy in which authority is used exactly as it should be in the service of organizational tasks. Leaders make decisions on behalf of the organization. They know, as do their followers, both the roots of their authority and its limitations (Obholzer 1994). All are clear about how to take up their roles. All are clear about the relation of those roles to one another and to the organizational tasks that anchor and link them.

Consistent disruptions of such authority relationships signal the intrusion of irrational elements into organizational life. This irrationality manifests itself in two primary, recognizable ways that derive their power from people's unconscious wishes to move both toward and away from authority, just as they once longed for both attachment to and separation from parental figures (Smith & Berg 1987; Wells 1985). The two irrational patterns of organizational authority represent the two sides of that equation, split off from one another. In one, leaders are authoritarian. Cut off from the roots and limits of their organizational authority, they believe and act as if they are omnipotent (Kets de Vries & Miller 1985; Obholzer 1994). Followers surrender their own authority, acting as if they are powerless, the better to be taken care of by the authority figures for which they long. In the second, leaders abdicate their authority. They and other organization members act as if they exist outside rather than within hierarchies. People become friends, create seemingly democratic decision-making systems, seek absolute consensus, and in other ways distance themselves from authority. In doing so they abandon the work itself (Hirschhorn 1997).

Pulls toward irrational authority patterns

These two patterns represent ways for individuals – and writ large, groups and organizations – to manage the unconscious tension between longing for and pushing away authority. One side of the polarity is repressed, the other embraced. The result is some form of disturbed culture of authority, which prevents organization members from working together as effectively as they might. This dynamic is not limited, of course, to caregiving organizations. In these organizations, however, there are certain factors that exert particularly strong pulls on members and leaders to maintain irrational patterns of authority.

Absorptions

I previously described how the experiences, emotions, and needs of careseekers are absorbed into caregiving organizations via their relationships with caregivers. Part of what gets absorbed is careseekers' experiences of dependency. These experiences are, typically, double-edged. There is regression. Careseekers long to be taken care of. They wish to be held tightly, as parents hold their infants and young children, and made safe and secure. Students want teachers to make their struggles to learn disappear. Patients want nurses, physicians, and therapists to heal them and make their pain go away. Congregants want their clergy to enfold them within a spiritual cloak that will shield them from the pain of loss, uncertainty, and death. The homeless, indigent, abused, and addicted want agency workers to fix them or their circumstances, leaving them whole and happy. Such longings are deeply seated. They are powerful, often unconscious; they drive careseekers toward a certain kind of help, and toward their own helplessness.

There is the other part as well. Careseekers bring with them an equally deep-seated desire to move away from the ministrations of others. They wish to fight, or to flee. Students may resent teachers, striking up rebellious stances, or they may withdraw from them, seemingly immune to their efforts to engage. Patients may be frustratingly non-compliant, arguing with their caregivers, missing appointments and medications, and in other ways refusing to cooperate. Congregants may attend services only occasionally, support their churches and clergy sparingly. The homeless, indigent, abused, and addicted may treat those charged with their welfare badly, pushing away their help, acting abusively, or running away altogether. The deeply-felt unconscious longings here, to not need others, are as powerful as those to need others. Careseekers wish to push away, and push away from, their own dependence and from those upon whom they are dependent (Memmi 1974).

Caregiving organizations absorb these wishes, and with them, careseekers' struggles with authority and dependency. When they are without settings in which they can examine these wishes for what, and whose, they really are, organization members take them as their own. The organization becomes the stage on which the struggle is enacted. Irrational patterns of authority are created when members suppress one wish and play up the other: they completely accept seemingly all-powerful leaders or completely resist seemingly untrustworthy ones. For their part, leaders act irrationally when they become the ultimate caregivers for their organizations, or when they abdicate completely the role of providing for others. Rational patterns of authority are created when members and leaders each hold on to both the wishes to embrace and limit organizational authority.

Individuals are drawn to irrational or rational patterns of authority by their own personal histories. People have internal models of authority: unconscious assumptions that dictate how individuals assess and act within authority relationships (Kahn & Kram 1994). Individuals with dependent models, for example, maintain an ongoing deference to authority – one's own and that of others – at the expense of using their personal authority to help guide their work, while those with counter-dependent models struggle to topple or deny the existence of an organizational authority structure, at the expense of work relationships and systems. People may also have partially unmet needs for good enough parenting: caregivers carry with them their own longings and resentments that make them particularly apt receptacles for the longings and resentments of others (Dartington 1994). Irrational authority relations are thus shaped by the absorption process, in which the needs and wishes of careseekers and caregivers mix freely and are acted out within the work context.

Collusions

A particular type of collusion between leaders and members often marks irrational authority patterns in caregiving organizations. Organizational members, caught up in longings to be taken care of, act as if their leaders are omnipotent. It is tempting for leaders to fall in with that demand and act as if they are more knowledgeable and powerful than they actually are. They create "a reciprocal relationship . . . which confirms the inadequacy of the one party and the superiority of the other" (Miller 1993: 227). Such relationships are reinforced by mutual projection systems. Subordinates vest by projection the competent parts of themselves in their leaders. They then act as if their projections give them the right to expect their superiors to make decisions for them (Lyth 1988). The leaders, for their part, vest by projection the irresponsible parts of themselves in their subordinates; by accepting the projections of themselves as responsible, they accept subordinates' responsibilities. "It is almost impossible," writes Miller (1993: 229), "to be the linchpin of a dependency structure without being seduced at times into illusions of omnipotence and omniscience."

Such seductions may be woven into the underlying cultures of caregiving organizations. Relations between caregivers and careseekers exert a natural pull toward a split between powerful and powerless, strong and weak, healthy and sick. Patients, clients, and students pull for those who care for them to suppress any doubts or fears and act as if they are all-knowing, in order to allow for the fantasy of some omnipotent other to free them of pain and problems. Physicians, teachers, ministers, and therapists are all pulled to be sorcerers and magicians, grand healers in the tradition of the medicine man (Guggenbuhl-Craig 1971). If they collude with those pulls, caregivers split the archetype of the healer/patient, creating a polarity between the regressed patient and the superior caregiver. Careseekers thus shed responsibility for their own development. Caregivers, seduced more or less willingly, become enshrouded in their own beliefs of omnipotence. They cannot then stimulate others to take up their own personal authority to learn, grow, or heal.

The seductions of caregivers by careseekers often help to create parallel authority relations between organization leaders and members. Caregivers look to their leaders as longingly as careseekers look to them. When leaders accept this and believe in the illusion of their omnipotence, irrational patterns of authority take root. Leaders may become benevolent rulers. They provide all resources, doling them out to their subjects as they see fit. They create visions, develop strategies, decide on courses of direction, and inform others of what they need to do to. Members follow along, using little personal authority to deviate from, question, or alter their leaders' plans. Conversely, leaders may become malevolent despots. They withhold resources, impose taxes and penalties, imprison some members, and cast off others. Members may flee, seeking safe havens inside or outside the organization. Or they fight, directly, with whatever weapons they can gather, or indirectly, through passive, bureaucratic rebellion. Each of these scenarios is rooted in the collusion between leaders and members to act as if the former is all-powerful and the latter powerless. Irrational authority patterns occur when organizational cultures accept such collusions as normal.

Irrational authority patterns are fueled by social defenses, created to ward off anxiety. Hirschhorn (1997) notes that threat and risk mobilize fantasies about authority figures, surfacing forgotten feelings of dependence. Freud (1959) described a dynamic in which group members project their own capacities for thinking, decision-making and personal authority onto the person of the leader. They disable themselves in return for the illusion of security. The leader is expected to look after, protect, and sustain members (Bion 1961). The same dynamic occurs at the organizational level of analysis. Members huddle together, metaphorically, beneath their leaders, in whom they invest awesome power to save them from whatever threatens. Such huddling may be episodic and temporary, or it may, over time, become woven deeply into the underpinning of an organization's culture.

The choice of dependence

The disruption of healthy patterns of authority at work represents the loss of collaborative work across hierarchical groups. There is also loss of the appropriate roles through which people interact. Mostly, there is the loss of primary tasks. Irrational authority patterns involve substitutions for primary tasks. People move away from assuming appropriate authority relative to one another, and thus avoid the anxiety of holding themselves and others accountable. Instead, they enact versions of a parent-child relationship. In some versions, members' needs for security, growth, and hope are met, and in others, they are continuously frustrated. In each version the meeting of members' own needs subsumes the primary task of meeting careseekers' needs, as members seek to avoid anxiety and accountability.

This process represents a choice on the part of organization members. The choice is often unconscious but a choice nevertheless. As Memmi (1974: 75) writes, "If the dependent perseveres in her slavery, it is because she more or less consents to it. She could throw off her chains, or at least lighten them considerably, if she really wanted to. Dependence is as much complaisance as deficiency." When organization members relate to their leaders as subjects relate to benevolent or malevolent rulers, they are implicitly choosing to do so. In caregiving organizations, of course, the choice may be over-determined, given the nature of their work. These organizations routinely struggle with the split between taking care of and supporting the growth and autonomy of careseekers (Lyth 1988). Not too little and not too much of the former must occur to support the latter. Institution members are at risk not only of getting too caught up in meeting others' dependency needs but of modeling their own relations with one another on a similar model of authority relations. I illustrate this process through the extended example of a church-affiliated children's hospital whose staff and leaders were struggling with authority relations.

New Hope Children's Hospital

The Catholic Church started New Hope Children's Hospital as a home for convalescent children of the poor. The facility was initially designed to accommodate 150 children whose severe physical and emotional conditions required long-term care and treatment. The hospital later reduced its bed capacity to 100, and was licensed to operate 40 pediatric medical/surgical beds, 40 physical rehabilitation beds, and 20 child/adolescent psychiatric beds. A board of directors representing consumers and advocates, the Catholic Church, and the lay and business community governed the hospital. The hospital remained under the auspices of the Catholic Church. It had developed a reputation for treating children with multiple disabilities and was regionally recognized for its expertise in treating children with special needs.

The hospital offered an array of programs and services. As the largest pediatric rehabilitation hospital in its region it dealt with both medical and psychiatric conditions. There were three inpatient programs: an acute medical/surgical and pulmonary service; pediatric and adolescent physical rehabilitation; and an inpatient children and adolescent psychiatric program. The hospital also offered three residential treatment programs for children with behavioral problems: a residential assessment program for evaluating children; an acute residential treatment program that served as an alternative to inpatient care; and a transitional care program for children who lacked suitable discharge placement options. A separate unit in the hospital also served the needs of children and adolescents who suffered from a combination of medical, developmental, and psychiatric disabilities. The hospital was organized around various departments that serviced its units and programs.

The hospital's organizational structure established the board of directors as the nominal authority, operating on behalf of the Catholic Church. The board authorized the president and chief executive officer (CEO) to run the organization. He was supported by a group of senior managers which included the medical director, chief operating officer (COO), chief financial officer (CFO), and the vice-presidents of plant engineering, rehabilitation, clinical and ambulatory services, marketing and development, finance, human resources, and admissions. The senior managers all had in turn a number of program/unit directors and managers for whom they were responsible. This latter group was considered middle management. They in turn directed the efforts of the hospital's relatively large medical, rehabilitative, nursing, educational, and support staff.

The CEO's involvement in New Hope began when he was president of a company that provided a certain service to financially troubled hospitals: cutting costs, downsizing staff, reducing services, and developing a sustainable financial strategy. He was asked by the New Hope board of directors and the then CEO to help the hospital climb out of its huge financial hole. Over the course of the next several years he helped stem the tide of financial losses at New Hope. There were lay-offs and strident cost-cutting measures. Managers and staff took pay cuts, agreeing to work for less money in order to keep various services and programs afloat. The board of directors rewarded the management company headed by the CEO with a long-term contract to operate the hospital. He agreed to the contract on the condition that he become the new president and CEO, while still maintaining an active consultation practice. He installed several members of his management company as vice-presidents of New Hope. This effectively blurred the boundaries between those who worked for him and those who worked for the hospital.

The history of the CEO as the savior of the hospital profoundly shaped the use of personal and organizational authority by him, the senior managers, and the middle managers. The relationships among the three groups were marked by a complicated set of dynamics surrounding the use of such authority. I learned of these dynamics in the context of a consultation with the hospital which was marked by three phases.

Lighting the candle, cursing the darkness

In my initial meetings with the COO, my primary contact at New Hope, she indicated that her goal was for the middle managers to become empowered to the point that they were able to initiate and implement innovative solutions. I agreed to help on the condition that I also work with senior managers, who had the potential to support or undermine such empowerment. We established three objectives for the consultation: to enable middle managers to assume more responsibility and initiative in the management of the hospital; to engage middle managers in the process of retaining staff; and to facilitate collaborations between middle and senior managers. I briefly met with the CEO, whose primary stated interest was training middle managers. He believed that the middle managers were unskilled in the budgetary and financial matters he thought necessary for them to more forcefully manage their areas.

I began working with the middle managers through a series of leadership development workshops. The middle management at New Hope existed less as a group than as a set of loosely connected heads of hospital units, programs, and departments whose attentions were focused downward, on their units, or upward, on their respective senior managers. The first session focused on the nature of their managerial roles. The session was intended to bring together the middle managers and begin to build them as a group. Several senior managers (including the COO) attended, which undermined the creation of a safe place for the middle managers to speak freely with one another. Attendance was mandatory for the middle managers. They had received a rather stern memo announcing the workshop and informing them that they needed to be present or have a written excuse. Those attending dutifully signed their names on a sheet at the back of the room when they walked in.

For much of the first part of the meeting the middle managers were mostly silent. The group allowed one member, the director of the dietary and house-keeping unit, to speak on their behalf. He was challenging and belligerent, and set himself up as the expert in matters related to leadership and management. The group used him to express their collective resentment against authority, which in this case was represented by an outside expert. Their resentment was expressed in other ways as well. One woman sat writing a letter. A second worked with a calculator and columns of figures. Yet another dozed, her eyes mostly closed behind her spectacles. With such acts they wordlessly communicated their resentment and anger, filling me with those feelings toward them. They wished, in this first session, to replace or ignore me and whomever and whatever I represented to them.

The managers worked in small groups to identify the problems they collect-ively faced. Each group focused on some version of the same problem: staff-ing. Many staff positions throughout the hospital were unfilled as people left and were not replaced; this placed a greater burden on those who remained, including the managers themselves, to chip in and do the work. Beneath the issue of staffing was that of retention. Young nurses, therapists, technicians, and other caregivers came to the hospital for training and then left for hos-pitals located in the larger urban area a few miles away, where they received more money and benefits. One manager quoted a figure of 50 percent staff turnover during the preceding three years. The middle managers were discouraged. They found it difficult to train people and have them constantly leave. The disruptions in care were also difficult for patients.

The group identified a number of obstacles to retention. Some concerned resources – money for higher salaries, benefits, advertising. Others were related to the lack of cross-training, mentoring, team building, and appreci-ation. The group was uncertain about its ability to influence this second set of factors, by creating environments in which staff members were getting their developmental needs met reasonably well. They could, of course, best do this by joining with one another. They could share resources, support, and ideas. They could develop and implement solutions together. There was much that they could do together, if they chose, that they could not do in isolation. They had for the most part not made that choice.

The second session occurred a few months later. No senior managers attended. The group began to engage with one another, with one woman asking everyone to introduce him or herself. Many did not know one another. It had been years, since before the financial crises that brought in their current CEO, that they had had the opportunity to talk with one another. Their only meetings had been with the CEO, who allowed them to ask questions and receive information. Those meetings were sparsely attended – the middle managers felt devalued and mocked when they asked questions, treated more as students than as colleagues – and had died out without fanfare. None, save the annoyed CEO, regretted their absence.

This second session focused on creating a process by which middle managers might identify and work together on a meaningful project related to staff retention. The purpose was for them to begin to create a culture of retention. Such a culture had yet to emerge from the senior management; it was left to the middle managers to create it. To do so they would have to first forge for themselves a network, a largely invisible web beneath the surface of the formal organizational structure. They could do so in the context of creating and implementing a project together. They would have to assume responsibility for the stages of a change project: diagnosis, action planning, implementation, and evaluation. They would also have to work with senior managers, providing them with information, rationale for expenditures, and reports related to staff retention.

The middle managers struggled with this idea. Their initial reaction was cynicism. They expressed this in many ways: they did not trust the senior managers to listen to them. The senior managers withheld power. They withheld information. They withheld support and appreciation. Any project, said the middle managers, would not lead anywhere. They would again be disappointed. It would be a waste of time and energy in a place where both are scarce. They felt disappointed and powerless, and as they spoke I felt the same in relation to them. I laid out their choices. They could simply stop, disband, and go back to their work. They could go through the motions, acting as if they were trying to change their culture without really doing so. Or they could engage a change process seriously, and in doing so open themselves up to both hope and disappointment. One woman responded, saying the options were slightly different to those I offered. "We can do nothing and be frustrated and disappointed," she said, "or we can try something and get slapped down again." An older woman spoke up. "It's better to light a candle than curse the darkness," she said. Heads nodded. At that moment the middle managers made a choice, of sorts, to try and take up their authority.

In the remainder of that session and the next the middle managers identified projects that might help them create a culture of staff retention. They discussed developing a shared system by which to track employees and monitor their career paths, as well as developing a collective orientation and cross-training system. The middle managers described the problems that such systems could solve. The group was split in its beliefs about whether they could actually solve these problems. Some members were angered that they even had to do so, that the senior managers had left it to them. Others were furious that the senior managers left them with no authority, no power to make decisions, and felt dispirited, sure that they would inevitably be hobbled by the senior managers. Another sub-set of the middle management group attempted to drive the work, believing that it was up to them to develop and implement solutions, given that they were most directly affected by staff turnover. They would, they said, have to work as best they could, given the limits of their authority and senior management's ability and willingness to empower them.

Over the course of several months following those sessions the middle managers' efforts to work together on the issues they identified became diffused. A few individuals assumed the lead in organizing others, gathering information, and drafting proposals to take to the senior management team. Their efforts to engage the other middle managers were undermined by those who chose to remain helpless or angry in relation to the senior managers. The sub-set of middle managers that wished to seek their own empowerment and join together in order to negotiate terms with senior management was slowly worn down by their helpless or enraged peers. They grew tired of their largely unsuccessful efforts to exhort, cajole, and convince. The projects lost momentum between leadership development sessions, to the point that they finally stopped altogether. Collectively, the middle management group chose, through their actions, to remain stuck waiting, blaming and resenting the senior management while mourning their own helplessness. They let the candle go out, then cursed the resulting darkness.

Covert operations

A second phase of the consultation process involved the senior managers. The middle managers felt that they would not be empowered without a willingness on the part of the senior managers to relinquish control. In preparation for a retreat with the small group of senior managers, I interviewed each vice-president. Most felt helpless and powerless in relation to the CEO. They complained that he controlled everything that went on in the organization – payroll, headcount, marketing and development – under the banner of containing costs. They felt he was overly involved in the details of each department. They said that the CEO held them responsible for specific duties yet withheld decision-making authority over their budgets. Some members were frustrated and angered by their disempowerment. Others were resigned but supported the middle managers as best they could while placating the CEO. A few simply wished that they had more say, that the CEO would change, that empowerment would start at the top. The portrait of the senior management mirrored that of the middle management.

I met with the CEO and COO in preparation for the senior management retreat. I told them that both middle and senior managers were struggling to make the transition from the crisis mode that they had been in since the major fiscal crisis a few years earlier to a mode that allowed them to create more stable systems of communication, learning, and quality improvement. I noted that they were frustrated with the tightness of the controls and that they felt ready to take up more decision-making authority. I described how the middle managers did not feel that the senior managers were themselves empowered, which made it difficult for them to take seriously the possibility of their own empowerment. The CEO took issue with each statement. He argued that without crises people did not work very hard. He argued that the senior and middle managers were simply not trained or skilled enough to make decisions that required the financial basics. He argued that without crises, the senior managers would not act as if they were accountable. I suggested that they were caught in a self-perpetuating cycle: the CEO created crises and the managers responded with short-term fixes that did not allow them to own either problems or solutions, or to invent systems that would forestall future crises. They then waited for the next crisis. The CEO responded by blaming the senior managers for their lack of initiative and responsibility. He could not, or would not, perceive his own responsibility for their behaviors.

The senior management retreat was marked by the senior managers' collective inability to speak directly of their dissatisfaction with the CEO and the crisis-management mode that left them off-balance and disempowered. They spoke of such to me during the retreat, in side conversations and over meals, out of earshot of the CEO. The retreat agenda was twofold. One agenda, presided over by the CEO, was to review the development and fund-raising plan. The CEO provided a fundraising goal – one million dollars – and challenged the senior managers to develop a series of proposals for meeting that goal. He set a group reward: spending money for their planned night of gambling at a resort near the retreat center. The group dutifully engaged in the activity, brainstorming and presenting ideas for fundraising events, approaches to wealthy donors, and appeals to community foundations. There was little dialogue or disagreement over the ideas that were raised. It was, more than anything else, a performance, with the CEO playing director and the senior managers enacting a play that they knew would mean little once it concluded.

The second agenda was for the senior managers to reflect on how they worked together. The group allowed one member, the vice-president of human resources, to praise how well the group was working together. Other members did not disagree. They spoke of themselves in ways that they thought the CEO would like to hear, describing the group as collegial and engaged. One member, the recently hired director of nursing, spoke more plainly. She described the group as less collegial than territorial. She described an earlier session in which she saw the CEO as offering non-constructive criticism, from which the senior managers withdrew. Her comments hung there in silence until another manager publicly contradicted her. (He later apologized to her in private, saying that he felt he had little choice; it was as if he had seized the opportunity to prove his loyalty to the CEO by publicly betraying her.) The others remained silent, covertly observing the CEO to gauge his reaction. He too was silent.

The rest of the meeting was guarded. The group generated a list of factors by which to evaluate themselves as an effective senior management team but was then unable to use those criteria to actually evaluate themselves. Each criterion – role clarity, accountability, appropriate authority – was met with relative silence. They were more candid in smaller groups, away from the CEO, describing their frustration with their lack of authority. When they reconvened as a large group, the senior managers offered sanitized versions of their conversations, praising the CEO. Under cover of small groups in which individuals could not be singled out they had shared their wish that the CEO empower others. They were thus able to name some of the issues, speaking anonymously, but were unable to work with and solve them when that required their taking up personal authority and speaking for themselves.

At the same time the senior managers longed for rescue. During our initial interviews they filled me with their frustration and anger at the CEO. At the retreat they expressed their longing for help, telling me that I was there to intervene with the CEO. They constantly looked at me and grimaced or rolled their eyes during sessions when the CEO was dominating. The COO was quite articulate about her wish for me to change the CEO, to get him to back away and allow others to assume appropriate authority. The CEO himself had never authorized this agenda. It had not been part of my contracting process. Nevertheless, this was the secret mission they most wished me to accomplish: to change him, as if I were a shaman who could do so without his knowledge, or to remove him, as if I were an assassin. As an outsider I was invested with such magical powers. I was also expendable if I was captured and executed.

Suppressing the revolt

The third phase of the consultation process involved the management group as a whole. The task was for the middle managers, senior managers, and CEO to create a more effective working relationship. This occurred through a series of full management retreats. Citing lack of resources, the CEO had abruptly cancelled the middle management leadership development work-shops, leaving them with little opportunity to continue to develop themselves into an effective cross-disciplinary group.

I met with the CEO in preparation for working with the whole manage-ment group. He told me that he was increasingly frustrated with senior man-agers who did not understand that they needed to answer to him immediately when he asked for something. He said that he was thinking of firing those who did not respond to his requests. He was also starting to bypass the senior managers and go directly to middle managers to make things happen. He also mentioned, as an aside, that he was concerned that the newest member of the senior management team – the director of nursing, who had confronted him and the others at the retreat – did not seem to fit in well with the others and might have to be let go. During this conversation I told the CEO that I was increasingly aware that people wished for me to change his leadership style and that he and I had never contracted for that work. I asked if he was interested in doing so, in order to help people feel more empowered and thus assume more responsibility. No, he said, he was not. He said he was willing to let the COO be a more visible internal presence, such that she would be the focal point of the empowerment process. I suggested that would work to the extent that they worked as a team and that he fully authorize her to take on that role without interference. He agreed.

The first full management retreat began with the managers examining the communication processes between the three groups, using the strategic plan as an example. It became clear that the CEO and COO had never clarified the process by which the managers ought to respond to their strategic plan. The senior managers were left to their own assumptions and preferences. Some never distributed the plan to the middle managers. Some held meetings to review and discuss it. A few made it available to others and never followed up. Some middle managers received the plan, others did not. Some responded to their vice-presidents on matters about which they cared, others ignored the plan entirely. There was no set process for input or feedback about the plan. This left everyone frustrated. The CEO and COO felt that no one was assuming any responsibility for the planning process, the senior managers were left waiting for the announcement of a formal process for their input, and the middle managers were upset by the inconsistent opportunities for input across departments. The strategic planning process offered a transparent example of the inability of the management group to work effectively across hierarchical boundaries.

Rather than proceed with our agenda and examine the underlying factors that had led to the dysfunctional process, and then create a more functional process, the CEO abruptly altered the course of the retreat in order to respond to what he felt were more urgent fundraising issues. He presented the list of fundraising ideas generated at the senior management retreat, complete with projected income and costs. As he moved through the list the attentions of the middle and senior managers drifted. Some looked beseechingly at the COO, others at me. The presentation complete, the managers dutifully broke into small groups and generated ideas for raising more money. The CEO read aloud the suggestions to the assembled group. He then handed them to the already overwhelmed development and fundraising department for implementation. The first retreat was over.

The second full management retreat opened with middle and senior management responding to the vision statement. They first worked in small groups. The CEO left while they worked and did not return. Most of the groups chose to focus on the retention issue. The final group suggested a process that involved creating a representative group whose task would involve collecting and analyzing staff input, developing ideas to enhance retention, and working to implement them. People offered ideas about how to construct the retention committee. They agreed to create the committee, schedule meetings, and report on their progress at the next full management meeting. The meeting ended soon thereafter, with the COO telling the managers that she thought the meeting was a useful beginning to a healthy process of input and empowerment.

I later met with the CEO and COO, ostensibly to plan the third retreat. Instead, the CEO told me that he was suspending the leadership development work. There was a financial crisis, he said. The hospital needed to find an extra four million dollars in its budget or through fundraising to make up for reduced payments from insurance companies and state agencies. He told me that a letter had gone out to all staff, telling them about the shortfall and how the hospital was dangerously close to the edge, lay-offs were possible, and that they would have to drastically cut costs and raise funds. He said that the board might press for the lay-offs, and that the prudent course of action was for him to cut jobs and programs, but that he would try to save them and that the staff should be grateful. The upcoming retreat would have a new agenda: management would have to help figure out what to do to save their jobs and those of their staff members.

The CEO also informed me that he had polled the senior managers and that they did not see any problems in how they were functioning in their work with one another, with him, or with the middle managers. He restated his original position that all that was needed was for the middle managers to get more training, so that they knew more about managing their budgets. He stated as well that staff retention was not really an issue for New Hope. The full-time employees (FTEs) were at or over budget, he said, except for a few areas in nursing; it was more a matter of a lag in people's perceptions, which had not yet caught up to reality. He asserted that morale was really quite good among the staff, as evidenced by people attending the staff/management parties. The senior managers had assured him that any issues were really a matter of "a few squeaky wheels." Finally, he said that he did not see the need for any representative committee, and that he would leave to the human resources department whatever retention issues that might need to be examined. Throughout, the COO sat mostly silent, unwilling to confront the CEO. Later, in her office, she told me that she had given up, that she had seen that he had no intention of releasing his control over the senior managers. Our work together, she said, was over. The revolt had been suppressed.

Co-dependency

Co-dependent relations are created when people join with others to satisfy complementary, often unconscious needs (Scarf 1995). Addicts are often enabled by others, who satisfy their own needs for control by unconsciously feeding the addicts' unhealthy dependencies; they become co-dependent, each needing the other to reaffirm a crucial identity. The New Hope management and CEO were co-dependent. They created a relationship in which the managers sacrificed their personal and organizational authority in return for the illusion that their CEO would save them from forces – competitors, insurance companies, the market – that threatened to destroy them. The CEO, for his part, sacrificed his ability to get support and collaboration from others in return for the illusion that he was New Hope's ultimate leader and savior. He assumed all personal and organizational responsibility, on behalf of all others; they assumed all the fear, longing, and anger, on his behalf as well as their own.

That was the deal the managers and the CEO struck. It proved ironclad in the face of covert attempts to break its terms. There were parts of the system that resisted the culture of dependency that sprang up around the CEO. Some middle and senior managers wanted to collaborate across hierarchical lines. They wanted to appropriately engage both their organizational authority to make decisions related to their roles, and their personal authority to develop innovative solutions to pressing problems. They were, however, overwhelmed by the culture of dependence. The culture was propagated at two levels: by senior managers unable to stop helplessly waiting for the CEO to change, or constantly enraged by his failure to do so, and by middle managers unable to stop helplessly waiting for their senior managers to change, or constantly enraged by their failure to do so. The helplessness and rage led to the same outcome, a disengagement that left people unable to collaborate with others to exercise authority. The senior managers were particularly disengaged from the exercise of authority. They did not exist as a group. They were thus unable to act as a buffer between the CEO and middle managers, and were respected by neither.

It might be said that followers often get the leaders for whom they wish. New Hope managers got a leader whose style, personality and needs led him to manage through fear and anxiety. The wish for such a leader was presumably rooted in the culture of their organization. That culture was related to the Catholic Church. Catholicism offers a certain template for leadership: the savior who takes the sins of the believers unto himself and is sacrificed on their behalf. The culture of dependence at New Hope fitted that template (which was unconsciously reinforced by the crucifixes adorning the walls). Another template was that of a hospital. The managers absorbed staff and client dependencies, and were primed to act out that dependency within their own authority relations. They thus colluded with the CEO's notion that he, not they, held the knowledge and skills, much like a New Hope physician in relation to disabled patients.

Such collusion enabled the propagation of New Hope's social defense system. Members joined together to create a dependency-oriented culture whose purpose was to keep at bay anxiety. The anxiety was multiply layered. On the surface, it was related to the hospital's survival in a difficult financial climate. Beneath the surface was anxiety related to the work the hospital did with a population of children and adolescents suffering severe physical and emotional disabilities. To witness that suffering, first-hand as a caregiver or second-hand as an administrator, was to experience pain. It was to experience fear that such suffering might well occur to oneself or to one's children. It was to experience much else as well: guilt and frustration, that one could not do more; shame, that one felt relieved to not suffer in such ways; anger, at the injustice of childhood disabilities; and longing, for miracles and cures.

New Hope's social defense system allowed managers to experience such emotions in relation to one another rather than to their clients. These emotions were real, and they needed expression, as steam needs escape from a boiling kettle. New Hope members had no place to engage in such expression. So they staged a play, whose plot would let them experience and express these emotions in a different, psychologically safer, context. The play was their organizational lives. Managers felt fear for their jobs. They felt guilty and frustrated that they could not do more for their staff. They felt ashamed at their relief that it would be staff that would be downsized. They were angry at, yet longed for, hierarchical superiors. And they felt the pain of being powerless, unable to change a situation that was unhealthy but seemingly immutable. These emotions and the play that allowed their expression were quite real to New Hope managers. The process served important functions for them, enabling them to express their reactions to others' suffering without having to confront those experiences more nakedly.

The consultation was suppressed when it threatened to disrupt the play. The COO and other managers chose to remain silent rather than speak up. The CEO reasserted himself as the crisis manager, akin to the leader of a military junta who, having taken power in a coup, does so again when the political regime threatens independence. I was expunged, the COO quietly withdrew her support for the covert rebellion, and martial law was reinstated. New Hope's social defenses remained securely in place.

The courage of self-authorization

In resilient caregiving organizations, members consistently struggle to authorize themselves personally and organizationally amidst the gravitational pull toward overly dependent relations. In organizations such as New Hope Children's Hospital, whose social defenses depend on members not assuming authority, this takes a great deal of courage. Managers risked their jobs when confronting the CEO. They risked being set up by colleagues who wished to prove their loyalty by pushing forth others as disloyal. They risked leaving their own departments and units vulnerable to downsizing and other forms of retaliation. In New Hope's culture of fear, asserting one's organizational authority (i.e., making decisions appropriate to one's role) or personal authority (i.e., speaking the truth of one's organizational experience) carried penalties most were unwilling to risk.

The culture was propagated by the managers' inability to join together. Middle and senior managers were relatively isolated, within and between their groups. Each manager was alone, left to deal with the CEO by him- or herself, and thus constantly on the defensive. Systemic change occurs when people join together. They share and examine their experiences, develop visions about what their organization could be and do, and mount campaigns to make it so. Such work involves members creating holding environments with and for one another. If the New Hope middle managers had been able to construct a holding environment for themselves, they might have authorized themselves as a group to create – to demand and work for – collaborative work relations with the senior managers. Similarly, if the senior managers had been able to construct a holding environment for themselves, they too might have authorized themselves to confront the CEO and assume authority on behalf of their tasks. For both groups, holding environments would have ideally led to a collective reflection on the play – of healer and disabled, savior and saved – that they were staging, and the underlying anxieties propelling that play.

In practice, this means that middle and senior managers each must create regular forums in which to meet and share problems, develop solutions, and seek to understand the nature, sources, and meanings of their stress. These forums allow for the creation of understanding: of managers' own experiences, of the caregivers they supervise, and of the larger covert play that they may be staging. People must create such forums for themselves, not wait for their leaders to do so for them. At New Hope, the middle and senior manager groups each needed to meet by themselves. They needed to talk of how their preoccupation with the CEO, and their de-authorizing of themselves to conform to his wishes, were harming their work, their collaborations, their satisfaction, and ultimately, their abilities to serve their patients. Such conversations ought not simply contain self-pity or complaint, or frustration and anger. People ought to focus on comprehending why they have created ineffective patterns of behavior, as managers, colleagues, and subordinates. Such comprehension lays the groundwork for concerted action on important tasks.

At New Hope, then, the middle managers would have convened themselves, pushing forward on projects they knew to be critical. Those able to do this would speak of the stress that they and their staff felt, of the lack of support from a senior management that attended too closely to the CEO and his wishes. They would acknowledge that their own strategies – staking out their own territories, withdrawing, placating their managers without asserting what they knew was in the patients' best interests – were unproductive and draining. They would develop a different strategy, of authorizing themselves to tackle pressing problems that affected them all. They might divide into smaller groups, each tackling a dimension of staff retention or training. They would define problems, gather information, create pilot programs and small experiments, implement them, and learn from what occurred. They would ask the senior managers for specific help and enlist their protection. They would not wait to be told to engage in such projects. They would assume it as part of their duties as managers, building the case for their own reasonable authority bit by bit until the rest of the organization accepted and expected it. For their part, senior managers would help and protect their subordinates, making the case when questioned that the projects were in the hospital's best interests. And they too would meet regularly as a group. They would work on minimizing the obstacles that the middle managers discovered in their work. They would reflect on their own experiences as a source of information about the hospital and its work on primary tasks.

This process puts both middle and senior managers in an organization such as New Hope on an admittedly risky path. When leaders such as the New Hope CEO are invested in certain arrangements of authority, it is dangerous for members to question those arrangements. They could be fired, isolated, publicly sacrificed in some fashion. They would need to plan their work carefully, in the way of any covert insurgency. This means understanding precisely the interests, styles, and points of leverage of those in charge. At New Hope, the middle and senior managers would need to frame their arguments in terms indicating the financial soundness of their ideas. They would need to speak the language of cost savings, enhanced publicity, and fundraising. And they would have had to enlist the protection of the COO, who would have to take a more assertive stance in her relations with the CEO. She might be able to do this if she had the sense that she was not alone, that others would rally around her when the CEO lashed out in response. In a system whose leaders protect themselves by dividing and conquering others, survival becomes a matter of not allowing such divisions to hold sway.

The courage of self-authorization is thus about people consciously making risky decisions that leave them vulnerable. Most of the middle and senior managers at New Hope chose to go along with rather than take on a CEO who they knew was, at some fundamental level, misleading the organization. They kept their jobs. They were not isolated or cast out. They suffered in a different way: they were aware of their own powerlessness, their inability to protect others whose work on behalf of patients was constantly interrupted by the CEO's crisis-oriented leadership. The managers lived with that awareness, and the guilt, frustration, and sadness it engendered. They preferred it to the alternative, which was to enforce the boundaries necessary for people to work effectively. New Hope's social defenses did not allow for such boundaries. They were routinely violated, most prominently at the top. The CEO intruded upon others as he wished. He went directly to middle managers to give them assignments. He arbitrarily changed agendas. He entered and left meetings without warning. Such intrusions and their silent toleration guaranteed that he would remain the central figure in the institution – the figure upon whom prayers and curses would be showered – and that all others would be left helpless, powerless to stop that which afflicted them. Collectively, that seems precisely what New Hope members wanted, albeit unconsciously.

The courage to authorize oneself is the courage to examine how organizational patterns of authority serve potentially irrational functions. It is to examine authority patterns aware of one's own collusion. It is, finally, to join with others to make conscious choices about how to exercise organizational and personal authority on behalf of organizational tasks. This process entails risks to oneself and to others; without risk, there is little need for courage. It also marks the path toward appropriate authority relations that ultimately serve the needs of caregivers and careseekers alike.

Chapter 7

Divided they fall

Caregiving organization members typically belong to particular departments or units, each dedicated to some aspect of the organization's primary task. The groupings ensure the integrity of sub-tasks: hospitals use self-contained units to safeguard patients; schools maintain academic departments to reinforce the learning of specific disciplines; treatment centers operate through departments that enable the work and training of staff members. Organization members may also belong to functional areas or professional disciplines. Hospitals, for example, contain nurses, physicians, technicians, and administrators, each of whom has a particular perspective and task based on training and roles. Each unit, department, function or profession is pointed toward some aspect of the careseekers' needs. Physicians diagnose, medicate, operate on, and develop protocols for patients, while nurses attend to them, technicians transport them, and administrators create systems that attract and serve them more capably.

As described earlier, splitting caregiving organizations into smaller, relatively contained departments, units and functional areas risks splitting the careseekers themselves into similar pieces. When caregivers work with only specific parts of careseekers they risk perceiving them in terms of those parts. Patients are not simply diseases; students are not simply English speakers or mathematicians; treatment clinic clients are not simply drug abusers. They are complex individuals with many aspects to their selves. When they are attended to as such by willing caregivers, they are most likely to heal, grow, learn, and develop. This is difficult for caregivers to do when they are primarily responsible for some particular piece of careseekers, such as their kidneys, history lessons, drug intakes, or relationships with abusive parents. Caregivers must perform the difficult work of holding onto the specific parts of careseekers for which they are personally responsible while building and holding onto fuller understandings of, and relationships with, them as well.

This work is made easier by the integration of departments, units, functions, and professional groups. Together, members across these groupings can work with careseekers as more complex individuals. When nurses, physicians, technicians, and administrators share information about any one patient, they are likely to develop a fuller understanding of his or her needs and experiences. The patient is more likely to be worked with as an individual through the collective ministrations of the hospital staff. The process is akin to the piecing together of a jigsaw puzzle. Members bring together the pieces that they have, based on their training and experiences, and place them in relation to one another. What emerges, ideally, is a fuller picture of a care-seeker and more understanding of what she or he needs. Resilient caregiving organizations routinely enable such integration. Their members work across the boundaries that define their particular groups. They solve what Roberts (1994c) described as the problem of *dual membership*: individuals are responsible members of both specific departments and encompassing work units, without sacrificing one for the other.

Archipelagos

A certain type of intergroup geography marks disrupted or failed collaborations among groups within caregiving organizations. The organization resembles an archipelago: a group of islands spread thinly throughout a large body of water, as if deposited there by some volcanic eruption. Departments, units, functions, and professions are isolated unto themselves, spread further apart than is warranted. They are connected only at points, via particular individuals who span distances and more or less serve as conduits. Otherwise, group members look inwards. They identify more with their specific tasks and perspectives than with the primary tasks of their organizations. Indeed, they perceive their groups *as* the primary organization. Other islands are dimly glimpsed as peripheral to the primary work, which occurs in their own group, on their own island. There is little consistent interdependence. There is much balkanization, and it is often seemingly intractable.

These archipelagos are maintained by a set of dynamics within and between organizational groupings, each of which is described in more depth below. These dynamics include intergroup splitting and projection, setting up "boundary spanners," and troubled points of connection.

Intergroup splitting and projection

Group members splitting off unwanted parts of their own groups and projecting them onto other organizational groups maintain inappropriate distances between groups. Group members come to hold a certain set of beliefs about themselves and about members of other groups that keep in place their mutual distance. An operating unit's nurses, for example, may believe that surgeons are arrogant and insensitive. This allows them to maintain an image of themselves as caring and compassionate. At the same time, by believing that the surgeons care more about operating techniques and procedures than about patients, the nurses are able to locate somewhere outside themselves their unacknowledged feelings of guilt over hurting the patient in the natural course of their duties (e.g., drawing blood). For their part, the surgeons may consider the nurses overly involved with patients. This allows them to maintain an image of themselves as dispassionate and object-ive while locating the emotionally involved parts of themselves within the nurses. While such splitting and projection is an intrapsychic phenomenon, occurring within individuals, it is transformed into an intergroup process by the collective engagements of group members (Smith & Berg 1987). Groups become locked into unconscious roles in the larger set of intergroup relations (Stokes 1994).

Splits between groups are also driven by what does *not* occur within them. Groups often avoid examining issues that lead to conflict among their members. They act as if the conflict lies elsewhere, with external groups (Smith 1989). This process follows a certain sequence. First, a group's members project onto some other group a particularly disturbing set of characteristics or identity. Second, the group acts as if its own members do not themselves possess those characteristics. Third, the group treats members of the other group as if they are like that identity, and in doing so, ignore information that suggests otherwise. Fourth, the group maintains an ongoing conflict with the other group, based on their disparagement of those split off and projected characteristics. Any potential internal group conflicts over those characteristics are thus suppressed in favor of external group conflict. Relations between organizational groups are sacrificed on behalf of a certain kind of order within groups (Smith & Berg 1987).

Setting up boundary spanners

Archipelagos are also maintained by dysfunctional relationships between boundary spanners – individuals whose roles require them to represent their groups to other organizational groups. They are often heads of department, units or functional areas (Stokes 1994). When relations between groups are dysfunctional, relations between boundary spanners are, as both cause and effect, necessarily troubled. The projections that group members make upon other groups are doubly concentrated upon these boundary spanners. Department heads come to symbolize split off characteristics. Their relations with one another are thus quite disturbed, given that they occupy symbolic as well as task-related roles.

This is a multifaceted dynamic. Boundary spanners are set up, by dint of their visibility in organizations, to attract a concentration of projections. Like lightning rods, they attract heat and energy, and absorb assaults while protecting others. They are heroic, after a fashion, but primarily they are casualties. "Intergroup conflicts," writes Stokes (1994: 128), "can easily provide scapegoats" who, while seemingly in positions of power, are particularly vulnerable to institutional pressures. Multiple parties set up these boundary spanners. Their own members, wanting to be led against other groups and requiring a leader strongly identified with "their" characteristics to do so, prop them up. They are set up by members of other groups, who require a visible target associated with the "other" identity and character-istics. They often cast themselves in their roles as well, led by unconscious needs to define themselves, and be defined by others, in relatively simplistic ways (Stokes 1994).

Boundary spanners may help maintain disturbed intergroup relations through their relationships with one another. Dysfunctional intergroup relations become locked within dysfunctional interpersonal relationships. The heads of the inpatient and outpatient departments of a treatment center are locked into an ongoing conflict whose origins no one recalls with certainty. Constant blaming, miscommunication and ill will mark the relationship between the head of hospital admittance and the head of nursing. The head of the teacher's union and the school headmaster wage a campaign against one another, using as weapons gossip and innuendo. Each of these disturbed interpersonal relationships maintains a dysfunctional intergroup relationship. Both sets of relationships – interpersonal and intergroup – remain disturbed as long as organization members maintain cover stories that simply blame boundary spanners themselves for the dysfunction. The more complicated reality is that the continued existence of the archipelago demands that those relationships remain disturbed.

Troubled points of connection

Archipelagos are also maintained by interactions between members of different organizational groups that leave them desiring distance rather than closeness. They rub up against one another in the course of their work and experience friction. Such friction manifests itself in various forms of conflict. Hospital administrators and physicians are at odds, each believing the other is making poor choices and sacrifices. Therapists and physicians disparage one another's approach to working with addicts. Science and art teachers argue over the place and meaning of standardized testing in the school's curriculum. Clergy members and church administrators cannot agree on the extent to which church members should be involved in planning events. It matters less what such conflicts are about than their implications for relations between the groups. When conflicts routinely leave group members upset with, disparaging of, and disconnected from members of other groups, it creates the conditions for continued intergroup splitting and projection.

Troubled points of connection are most apparent when members of different organizational groups try to work together. Interdisciplinary teams and task forces become the arenas in which group representatives play out relations between their groups. The interpersonal relations among the group representatives are locked, like guided missiles, into patterns determined by ongoing intergroup splitting and projection (Alderfer 1987). Organizational productions of one sort or another are shaped (or rather, misshaped) by group members' wishes to maintain distance from those defined as "other." At such points, when integration is imperative, individuals act in relation to one another in ways that maintain their dis-integration as an organization. This is particularly evident in the context of hand-offs of patients between hospital units, of students between academic departments, of clients between school and residential care. Such transitions are disturbed by and reinforce frictions between organizational groups.

The costly construction of safe havens

The archipelago exists primarily because it seems to create safe havens for group members. People retreat to their units – their work groups, departments, functions, and professions – and draw close to one another. Like combat veterans whose units are stranded in the field, they form fierce connections to one another; they draw support from one another, watch one another's backs, provide cover, and join with one another in the fight for survival against their enemies. They remain within their bunkers. There they cleave to one another as if it is only in the shelter of one another that they can survive.

These shelters are built at some cost. Unit members draw irrationally close to one another, suppressing internal conflicts that might otherwise cause discord but are ultimately useful to their work. They draw irrationally distant from members of other units, creating external conflicts that might not otherwise exist. Their sense of safety is thus built upon a tenuous foundation. They are able only to express their similarities, not their differences that might, if given space, flourish into useful conflict that would ultimately reveal them more fully to one another and hence create a more authentically safe environment for further self-disclosure (Jourard 1971; Smith & Berg 1987). To remain within their shelters, unit members must agree to simplify their worlds. They must act as if they are very much like one another and very much different from other organization members. They thus close off the possibility of authentic help from members of other units.

These shelters may be understood as social defenses. Unit members seek to defend themselves against the anxiety generated by their primary tasks. They simplify their emotional experiences in order not to deal with disturbing ambiguities, ambivalences, and other sources of emotional confusion. This simplification occurs along organizational fault lines that demarcate the islands of the archipelagos. Unit members split off what they do not wish to see within their selves and export it to other islands. Each island thus contains some part of the collective experience on behalf of the organization as a whole. Therapists empathize with the patient's history, childcare workers deal with the here and now of behavioral consequences. Nurses are compassionate, surgeons dispassionate. Clergy are idealistic, outreach workers eminently practical. These are partial truths. They are also simplifications that falsely divide complicated experiences and render them palatable. Members thus do not have to hold onto multiple truths. Specific emotions become associated with specific units, and locked within them. Unit members are thus spared internal struggles with emotional complexities. They are also spared the opportunity to examine, in concert with members of other organization units, their unvarnished experiences and what they signify about the careseekers and how best to serve their needs.

Greenvale Residential Treatment Center

The Greenvale Residential Treatment Center (GRTC) provided educational, residential and clinical services to approximately 100 at-risk boys with emotional and behavioral difficulties severe enough to interfere with their abilities to remain in their schools, homes, or communities. The clients, ranging in age from 7 to 18 years, typically had disorders that manifested in aggressive, withdrawn, or self-injurious behavior. GRTC staff worked with these clients in the context of three primary programs. A day school helped students improve academic and social skills, develop more appropriate behavior controls, and enhance self-esteem. A clinical department provided diagnostic evaluation, individual and group psychotherapy, and case management. A residential department oversaw various types of residential treatment facility. Three houses, containing short-term, acute clients or those who were in intensive programs related to sexual compulsion or fire-setting, ringed the main GRTC campus. There were also several off-campus houses located in surrounding communities, designed to prepare clients for successful transition back to their home communities. The residential program involved the creation of a therapeutic milieu, in which group interaction, behavioral control, consistent daily routines, and the teaching of appropriate social skills combined to support individual development.

The three departments – education, clinical, and residential – were each managed by a department head. The departments were both separate and integrated in their operations. The separation was geographical, with the activities of each department occurring in particular areas of the campus, and temporal, as clients moved from one area to another during their days and nights. The residential department was responsible for the clients before and after the school days and weeks, during which the education department was responsible. The clinical department was responsible for the clients at specific, relatively limited points during school days, when therapy, medication, or case management was required. Childcare workers staffed both residential and education departments; the latter also contained teachers certified in special education.

An administrative team oversaw the departments and ancillary services and set the strategic direction of the agency. The executive director worked with external constituencies in surrounding communities, state agencies, and other institutions charged with overseeing the successful placement of at-risk youth. The director of programs oversaw the daily operations of the residential and education departments. A director of clinical services supervised the operations of the clinical department, both therapy and case management services. The director of administration oversaw client movement into, through, and out of the agency. A business manager was responsible for the budget, accounts receivable and payable, and other financial aspects of the agency. These five administrators were collectively responsible for the agency. They in turn reported to a board of directors whose actual oversight was nominal.

I conducted an organizational diagnosis of GRTC over the course of six months, using observations and interviews, culminating in a series of feedback meetings with organization members (see Kahn *et al.* 2003). The themes presented below were part of the feedback material.

Pockets of support

GRTC existed mostly in the form of sub-groups. Members identified more with their departments, programs, houses, shifts, and informal cliques than with the agency as a whole. Various types of boundary between the groups reinforced their isolation. There were physical boundaries, as departments, programs, and houses were geographically distinct. There were temporal boundaries, given that staff had different work shifts, with the weekday staff rarely overlapping with night or weekend staff. There were the boundaries imposed by the ways in which departments worked with different aspects of clients: the education department focused on the intellectual, the clinical department on the psychological, and the residential department on the behavioral. There were cultural boundaries as well, by which departments and the cliques within them marked themselves with particular language, humor, and practices. These boundaries made it easier for group members to distinguish themselves from others and create pockets of support.

Staff members needed the support. They worked with emotionally troubled teenagers who acted out physically, assaulting staff and one another, and who occasionally needed to be restrained or put in isolation rooms. They acted out verbally as well, yelling obscenities or inciting their peers toward violence. Some acted out sexually, assaulting one another, while others were more covertly manipulative of one another and staff. Staff members worked in the face of such assaults daily. They talked of their work as if they were on the battlefield, members of MASH (mobile army surgical hospital) units charged with taking care of the angry wounded's emotional cuts. The resulting culture was shaped by the clients' anger and woundedness. Staff members mirrored the adolescents' instincts for survival and general mistrust of others. They created a culture they routinely described as "tough" and "negative." Members learned to care for and protect themselves, found selected others on whom to rely, or left the agency altogether.

Each department had a core group of staff that demonstrated commitment through their tenure, diligence, and hours worked. Members of these core groups helped retain facts, ideas, and practices that survived normal staff turnover. They knew who to go to for what, how to get things done efficiently, how to gain support for ideas and practices. They were the veterans, savvy about survival, and not all that willing to reach out to new recruits who had not yet proven themselves. The core drew together, creating bonds that sustained them in the face of difficult physical and emotional work. They created relatively isolated safe havens, finding shelters in their relations with one another. Those who were not able to latch onto such support did not last long.

The core groups were formed by people turning to those closest to them: others on their shifts, in their departments, with whom they shared similar perspectives. Childcare workers helped one another restrain physically abusive clients. Teachers helped one another stop situations from spinning out of control. Department members provided information to one another. Staff members were so spread out from one another, geographically and temporally, that it was easy for clients to manipulate them, playing them off against one another by telling them things that were not true and difficult to verify. The more information that staff members shared with one another the less susceptible they were to being manipulated by their clients. Such support occurred within the relatively tight boundaries that kept agency sub-groups separate from one another. This was most clear in the context of interdepartmental boundaries, which effectively carved up the agency. The residential, education, and clinical departments were islands unto themselves.

Interdepartmental disintegration

The promise of a therapeutic milieu is that daily interactions between clients and agency staff, regardless of specific context or task, are therapeutic (Hinshelwood 2001). When agency members created relatively safe havens for themselves, seeking protection against the violence emanating from their clients, however, they withdrew from integrating themselves on behalf of those clients. The education, residential, and clinical departments each pursued its own agenda. This was partly a function of disciplinary differences. Each department operated on a different set of principles rooted in a set of beliefs about what ultimately would best serve clients. They articulated shared goals but held different beliefs about how to achieve those goals. The educational department focused on behavioral outcomes. The clinical department focused on cognitive and emotional processing of past and present events. The residential department focused on teaching life skills and fostering peer relations.

While each of these foci were clearly integral to the ultimate development of GRTC's clients, the differing beliefs and premises translated into a struggle for which department (and corresponding treatment philosophy and practice) would be primary in the agency. Staff members routinely disparaged members of other departments. They blamed one another. Incidents would occur – a child ran away, another stole a van, a third brought drugs into the building – and staff members would immediately look to blame other departments. They were also routinely disrespectful to other departments' members. Rather than inquire about their experiences, perspectives, and approaches in specific situations, they circulated rumors or confronted them in a bullying or disrespectful fashion. Or they simply ignored one another. Teachers, childcare workers and therapists would not seek out one another to provide crucial information. Clients would suddenly erupt into violence, and staff members lacked the information necessary to put those actions in their proper context.

The lack of integration among the three departments was located most strongly within the relations between the three department heads. The system was designed on the premise that the heads would be the primary integrating mechanism. Ideally, they would confer, advocate, and struggle toward consensus as a daily practice. No judge was needed as long as the three heads acted in concert for the good of the agency and its clients. These conditions were not met; the triangle was notably unsteady. The clinical department head withdrew from the advocacy process, leaving the heads of the residential and educational departments to battle more publicly for prominence in the agency. These two women did so with a vengeance, taking every opportunity to weaken the other's stature. The agency was rife with rumors about their latest battles, waged publicly in administrative meetings and privately through back-channels. Their battles were treated largely as interpersonal – they simply "couldn't get along," or "hated each other." The education department head was widely perceived as "ambitious," and the residential head as "a bully." These women acted in ways that helped confirm such projections.

Led by their heads, department members were quite territorial in their relations with one another. In scrabbling for their own territory they neglected to maintain a common ground on which agency members could meet and work through issues. This was most obvious in the context of treatment teams. The teams were composed of representatives from each department who met together weekly to create and evaluate treatment plans for each client. These teams were poorly attended and poorly functioning. Members pushed their own department-based perspectives and agendas. They were often instructed by their department heads to protect departmental interests. Team members were often unprofessional, telling long stories that violated confidences, speaking rudely or aggressively to one another, and accusing rather than inquiring about one another. Resulting treatment decisions, to the extent that they were made, were not communicated throughout the agency. Staff members continued interacting with clients based on their own departmental perspectives.

The treatment teams were thus primarily settings in which departments could act out against one another in the guise of working on multidisciplinary treatment plans. There were no other cross-departmental settings; without agency-wide meetings and training, no other agency-wide forums allowed for meaningful dialogue. Each department was thus free to create its own culture, which inevitably existed in counterpoint to those created by the others.

The residential department, containing the most staff, had the strongest culture. It was marked by anger and resentment toward the rest of the agency. The residential staff – many of whom represented minority groups and were, compared to the teachers and therapists, relatively uneducated – felt unappreciated by the agency. Their department head fueled that perception. She routinely told staff of her grievances against the other departments and senior administrators, proclaimed her belief that the residential department was the most important in the agency, and continuously incited her troops with anger toward other departments and the administration. She also ensured that residential staff members who broke ranks and spoke well of or collaborated with those outside the department were punished, through shunning or assignment to undesirable shifts. The department remained isolated, its members joined in collective resentment and anger. Its members routinely acted out that anger through bullying and other intimidation tactics.

The education department was composed primarily of special education teachers. The department was steeped in the realities of attempting to educate clients for whom school was a trigger for feelings of inadequacy, inferiority, and anxiety. The teachers were generally realistic about the possibilities of their effectiveness with the students, steering between hopefulness and hopelessness. They tried to keep these extremes at bay, focusing on the immediacy of lesson planning and curricular reviews. The education department head was engaged with the administration in developing and striving toward educational goals. She presented herself as eminently reasonable, and in her relations with the other two department heads, as long-suffering and victimized. Her staff members did the same in relation to members of the residential and clinical departments, portraying the former as unprofessional and rude and the latter as overwhelmed and of limited use. This left them as the most reasonable and practical, simply trying to do their jobs amidst an unprofessional environment. They were largely cynical about the possibility of change in the agency's dynamics.

The clinical department was composed of trained therapists, mostly social workers who had or were planning to earn masters degrees, and case managers, who were newer to the field. Clinical department members were Caucasian and college educated, and regularly received case supervision. The department was marked by a lack of energy. Therapists rarely joined with one another, spending much of their time in their offices with clients. The case managers were off coordinating the movements of the clients into and through the agency and were relatively disconnected from other members of the department. The department was marked by a sense of lethargy. Department meetings, when they occurred, contained little energy. They were marked by the monologues of the department head, who rambled, skipping from one tangent to another, and only occasionally helping to connect department members to one another. The clinical department was constantly drowning in paperwork. Its members, and in particular the department head, seemed unable to get on top of their work. In this regard, they presented much like clients whose emotional states – anxiety, depression, and anger – prevented them from focusing on and completing specific, concrete tasks.

The cultures of the three departments were, in many ways, alien to one another. Unsurprisingly, this created inconsistency in their collective treatment of clients. A teacher might "consequence" a child for acting disruptively in class, putting him on isolation once he was back in the residence, but the residential staff might well reverse the consequence because they distrusted the teacher's motives and rationale. Or the residential staff might ask for support from teachers or clinicians in helping with the transition into the classroom and be rebuffed by teachers who said they needed to finish preparing for class. Such transitions – students leaving school for the residences, or on Fridays, for the weekend – were flashpoints. The three department heads sought to protect their staff from being "on the floor" during those times; each argued that their people needed to prepare, or do paperwork, or leave. Transitions routinely frayed interdepartmental relationships and upset clients already anxious about transitions.

Administrative team abandonment

This description of GRTC begs the question: Where were the senior administrators? The organizational diagnosis indicated that they largely abdicated from the work of managing the relations among the three departments. They did not provide a set of principles to guide department heads' advocacy and consensus. Nor did they serve as the ultimate arbitrator. The other members of the agency framed this absence as a form of abandonment and reacted variously with anger (residential), cynicism (education), and longing (clinical).

The lack of administrative presence was clearest when it came to what agency members most clearly and strongly longed for: accountability. Members of each department despaired about the senior administrators' inability or unwillingness to sanction inappropriate behavior from staff members toward one another or clients. Examples abounded. A weekend childcare worker forced a client to stand barefoot on a milk carton as punishment, with no major disciplinary action. Staff members yelled at one another, to the point of verbal abuse, with little repercussion. A residential supervisor forgot to pass out medications and was barely reprimanded. Reports of these and other infractions were routinely made to the senior administrators, and just as routinely resulted in little observable disciplinary action.

It was, of course, not simply that senior administrators were unaware of what staff required. There was the tight labor market, which seriously weakened administrators' power. There was also the fact that they were not, in practice, much of a team. The senior administrators, like other members of the agency, had created their own personal pockets of support and in doing so focused less on the agency as a whole. They did not meet as a unit *per se*, joining instead the department heads and other middle managers in an all-purpose (and largely ineffective) monthly meeting. Each of the five senior directors found other places of support outside the agency, in another department, or in an administrative sub-group. The senior administrative team did not exist as such, its members sliding out of the group to find support elsewhere. They abandoned one another as much as they did the rest of the agency. Privately, they reported feeling guilty about doing so.

The lack of accountability was also rooted in the psychology of the agency. Its stated mission was to create a safe, therapeutic environment for the clients; its mission, in practice, was sheltering clients, protecting them from a harmful world. Agency staff and administration created a home, of sorts, for their clients. They created one for the staff as well. It was the place of unlimited chances for staff members. Staff members were rarely fired. The agency had become a shelter for its own staff. People were taken in, provided with a steady job and a residence, and excused from full responsibility for actions that were not in the agency's and clients' best interests. There were lots of excuses and second chances for people, without much discipline or oversight. Administrators looked the other way rather than force staff to take responsibility for their actions.

In this context, the senior administrators were the protectors rather than the leaders, which would have required them to take up their legitimate authority and hold others, department heads and staff members alike, accountable. Their decision not to do so, while unconscious, was also rooted in the agency's implicit psychology. To assume a muscular authority at GRTC would be experienced as dangerous, given the wealth of abusive experiences that clients (and many staff) had in relation to such authority. Senior administrators largely chose not to become the focal points of a great deal of anger. They took up a softer, nurturing authority. They justified this in terms of shelters, the second chances that people deserved. To have done otherwise, to hold others justifiably accountable, would have unleashed a fair amount of rage that staff had "soaked up" from the clients. In the face of that possibility, the administrators melted away, from their roles and one another, and largely left agency members to their own devices.

Compelling distractions

The patterns of intergroup behavior at GRTC were not the fault of any one group or individual but represented an unspoken collusion among agency members more generally. The culture and practices of each group were strands that, woven together, created a tapestry of social defense. The disintegration of the agency into its groups served functions for the agency as a whole. The functions were both general and specific. At the general level, they enabled agency members to avoid experiencing anxiety related to trying to create a therapeutic environment for emotionally and psychologically damaged children and adolescents. The difficulty of that task – of repairing such damage with few resources, little time, and often unsupportive or hostile family networks – was large. So too was the potential depth of sadness, rage, depression, and guilt triggered by working with such a population. Agency members thus created within their organization a way to flee from examining their efforts and experiences. They did so by fighting among themselves. Their intergroup warfare was in fact a compelling distraction from troubling questions and painful emotions.

The splits between the groups also heightened their power to provide safe havens for their members. The more that departments, and the cliques within them, were at odds, the more forcefully their members pushed away from others and moved toward one another. The ongoing splits between the groups thus fed the momentum of people turning toward their own groups for support. This came at a price: members maintained the illusion that all flaws belonged elsewhere, in other groups, not in their own groups. People consistently blamed "others," ignoring the inappropriate or ineffective behaviors that occurred within their own groups.

The splits enabled agency members to avoid the difficult work of integrating information about, interpretations of, and experiences with, clients throughout the agency. The underlying model of a therapeutic environment honoring equally the role of each department is difficult to create in practice. It requires members to constantly communicate with one another. It requires them to first spend enough time with members of their own departments and programs to sift through their experiences with each client and come to a collective understanding of his or her issues and progress, and second, to represent that perspective in cross-departmental forums and interactions. GRTC possessed neither the slack resources – time, extra staff – nor the technology that would allow for such communications. The intergroup splits created not simply a shared distraction from enacting the agency's underlying model but a compelling rationale for avoiding doing so.

The absence, in practice, of an integrated therapeutic model left a void in the agency that was filled by the power struggle between departments. The department heads were territorial. They fought over scheduling. They fought over staffing patterns. They fought over the movements of clients into, throughout, and out of the agency. They fought for the sake of fighting, to impress upon one another their importance in the agency. Mostly, they fought on behalf of the agency, whose members collectively stood by and reinforced them in the manner of a crowd at a boxing match urging on its fighters. The collective, unconscious wish was that the program heads would fight until one remained standing; the agency would thus have a single champion whose focus (academic, therapeutic, or social skills) would cancel out the others and relieve them of the necessity of integration. At the same time, agency members unconsciously did not wish this to occur, for they knew it would be a destructive oversimplification. So they maintained a battle that could and would not end. When department heads grew weary of battling, agency members invariably sought them out, telling them, in so many words, how important their work was, how much their departments needed them to continue the struggle, how both staff and clients depended on them to win. The department heads would inevitably answer the bell, stumble out toward one another, and renew their battling.

The "program head" issue displaced other issues related to the difficulty of maintaining a generally supportive culture in the agency, reconciling healthy tensions across departments, and developing and enforcing administrative systems for effective teamwork. It provided such a compelling distraction that agency members were unable to step away from it and reflect upon how they were staging a re-presentation of client issues. They were thus unable to examine how they had unconsciously re-created the situations of many of their clients: abandoned by authority (i.e., administrators), isolated and depressed (i.e., therapists), frustrated and enraged (i.e., residential department members), and trying hard to succeed in a seemingly hopeless situation (i.e., teachers). Just as the families of their clients had done, they created scapegoats and filled them with pain, bullied and were bullied by one another, and dis-integrated into warring factions. This re-creation was a social defense, but also a collective, unconscious hope that the clients' experiences would be re-presented and worked with as such. They were not. Members remained stuck in an ongoing re-enactment of that which they imported from their clients.

Fueling this process was agency members' shared desires to simplify their painful emotional experiences at work. Members of each department were drawn to a particular emotion – anger (residential), sadness and longing (clinical), cynicism (educational), and guilt (administration). It was as if these emotions were deposited in separate departments, like vaults containing specific emotions. This simplified agency members' experiences greatly. Individuals did not have to struggle with the multiple, conflicting emotions naturally triggered by their work with their clients. Instead, they absorbed and contained specific emotions on behalf of others, who did the same for them. The struggles occurred externally, between departments, rather than internally, within individuals' psyches.

At the same time, the agency's culture favored one emotion over others. Agency members were constantly angry at one another. The dominance of anger over the other emotions was multiply determined. The residential department was the largest in the agency and its members gravitated toward frustration and anger, bringing the other parts of the agency with them. Further, anger is often easier to express and live with than sadness, longing, or guilt. Those emotions pull for people to withdraw rather than engage. The anger thus provoked and energized agency members. They were stirred to engage with one another, albeit not always productively. The culture implicitly sanctioned their expressing anger that, if directed at its source – the clients and their families, schools, and other parts of their communities that had abandoned them – would undermine their work with the clients. Their routine blaming of one another provided yet another compelling distraction from the more complicated experience of absorbing, containing, and working effectively with their clients.

Failures to collaborate

The story of GRTC is that of a series of failures to collaborate. Agency members did not inhabit the same organization but instead split into sub-organizations, each with its own task, perspective, and leadership structure. They maintained the divisions by acting as if members of other units were enemies. The definition of collaboration became skewed: individuals refrained from sharing information and support across departmental lines in order to not be branded "collaborators," traitors who aided and abetted the enemy and were summarily ostracized from their safe havens. When caregiving organizations splinter into warring factions – departments, units, task forces, programs, functions – members perceive one another as allies or enemies, and act accordingly. Meaningful collaboration across enemy groups is impossible.

Certain conditions create and maintain this state of affairs. First, organization members lack a shared primary task, clear and compelling enough to provide meaning and momentum for their identifications with (rather than against) one another. Primary tasks anchor people to one another. They provide the rationale for people to link arms with one another and form an unbroken boundary separating them from their environment while joining them together. Second, organization members lack places in which to examine the emotions that they absorb from their clients. If unit members cannot excavate and examine their emotions, they will both act them out and defend against them simultaneously. Inevitably, this will involve using other groups as foils. Third, there are failures of leadership. Unit leaders allow their groups to be too sealed off from others. Organization leaders allow dysfunctional intergroup relations to flourish. They enable social defenses to take the place of clear and compelling primary tasks.

These conditions create organizational vacuums. Groups fill them, like rogue military units loosened from their tethers by a military in disarray. The groups define their own purposes. These are related mostly to their own survival and defense. They act as if they need to defend against other groups, but beneath the surface they are defending against the array of emotions generated by their work. The ensuing struggles between units, each casting others as enemies, are members' collective attempts to struggle with the absence of clear and shared primary tasks. To gain clarity, they pit one version of the task against another in fights over resources, power, and priorities, hoping that their leaders will choose and resolve. However, since each unit contains a vital piece of the task, the struggles are doomed to continue unabated, such that no piece gets lost. The system remains in a steady state of dis-integration, the rogue groups claiming bits and pieces of territory from one another. Without the possibility of resolution they remain locked in stalemate.

This defensive process does disservice to both organization members and clients. Some organization members become casualties. Like the GRTC department heads they assume roles that require them to re-enact painful scenes, battling with one another or creating victims and victimizers. Locked into such roles, they cannot easily give or receive support to one another and are left isolated, containing various emotions for which there are few avenues for release. Their units are similarly afflicted. Unit members become locked into intergroup relations that prevent them from giving or receiving support across enemy lines. Certain emotions get associated with and locked into specific units, enabling members to feel some emotions (e.g., anger, sadness) but not others (e.g., joy, compassion) deemed the province of other units. All become casualties, in that they are forced into one-dimensional experiences. They play stock characters in the collective social defense, with little room for their more complicated humanity.

In such cases it is difficult for careseekers to be worked with as complex, three-dimensional individuals. Caregiving organization members who have simplified their own internal lives so as to only allow themselves specific emotions are less likely to be able to work with careseekers' full range of emotions. When one unit, such as the residential department at GRTC, contains and reinforces in its members a constant state of resentment and anger, they are less likely to enable their clients' own joy or sadness. When another unit, such as the clinical department, is steeped in sadness, its members may be less likely to enable their clients to express their rage. The clients themselves are thus unconsciously pushed to mirror the organization's dynamics. Like their caregivers, they must simplify their internal lives, expressing only certain emotions at certain times. They become "gifted children," in Alice

Miller's (1981) phrase, able to sense and produce the emotions and experiences expected of them, in order to produce only that which their caregivers can themselves handle. Like their caregivers, they become fragmented. As they move between units they call upon some parts of themselves and suppress other parts, the better to match their environments. Organizational dis-integration is matched by internal dis-integration, within careseekers and caregivers alike.

These dynamics can change only to the extent that organization leaders and members reconfigure boundaries within and between organizational units. Integration must occur at each level of the organization. It begins with senior management. At GRTC, the administrative team needed to create boundaries around itself: members needed to meet by themselves, without department heads, and examine their leadership practices and the implications for agency functioning. Ideally, this would involve their acknowledging their own flight from assuming authority as a group, and exploring why and how they had done so and at what costs to themselves and others. Once they began to join together – to identify themselves as the senior administrative team, with all that entailed – they would be able to hold themselves and others accountable. In particular, they could act jointly to intervene in the department head conflicts that distracted the agency from the work of integrating across all departments. This intervention would not simply involve removing one or more department heads. Rather, it would involve creating an integrated model of a therapeutic environment – its principles, practices, and disciplines – and holding the department heads and their staff accountable for its implementation.

This process demands the integrity of boundaries not simply around senior management teams but around middle management groups as well. The department heads at GRTC needed to create reasonable working relationships, given that they would inevitably model the nature of the integration, or lack thereof, between their departments more generally. They would also need to meet as a group, identifying and solving problems that arose in their attempts to implement a therapeutic environment. They would have to hold that space regularly, and use it well, to slowly move themselves and their constituents away from the conflict and disintegration that marked their relations and upon which the agency more generally depended as a social defense. This would involve a fair amount of reflection, enough to pause and then interrupt the habituated tendencies of department heads to blame and lash out against one another. They would need help with this work, from an administrator they trusted or an outside consultant.

Interrupting dysfunctional patterns throughout organizations more generally involves the ongoing creation of boundaries that maintain the integrity of their units. The lack of integration across units is driven partly by an inability of unit members to surface and work through conflict among themselves; it thus becomes exported across unit boundaries and fuels intergroup conflict. Halting such destructive processes requires unit leaders to create settings that enable members to work through their conflicts with one another. Such settings are marked by regular meetings, norms that support surfacing and discussing conflicts in constructive ways, and real accountability for not doing so. At GRTC, department heads would need to ensure that their members confronted one another over troubling issues and inconsistent practices with the clients rather than simply revert to the knee-jerk blaming of other departments' members. The department heads, held accountable by the senior administrators for integrated practices across the agency, would have to support the difficult conversations both within and across their departments.

The creation of appropriate collaborations across caregiving organizations thus depends on establishing regular settings in which unit members can address their own practices and experiences. Armed with insight and understanding, unit members can venture forth to integrate their work with that of other units. Collaborations, like relationships, cannot be truly healthy unless each party has the maturity to examine and develop their own behaviors separate from those of the other. In the context of such differentiation, people are not forced into simplified emotional experiences. In the context of such differentiation, integration may occur, as members turn away from battling one another and toward addressing the issues that affect them all. In caregiving organizations, this integration is crucial, not simply for staff members but for the careseekers who look to them as models for waging their own struggles to integrate their experiences as they heal, grow, learn, and recover.

Chapter 8

Teams, real and imaginary

Teams are ubiquitous in caregiving organizations, as elsewhere. There are teaching teams in grade levels, surgical teams in operating rooms, ministry teams for community projects, childcare worker teams, task forces for developing strategy and evaluating practices. Such teams complete tasks too complex for individuals. Properly designed, real teams are integrating mechanisms that draw people together and point them toward specific, unifying goals. Improperly designed, they are groups masquerading as teams. Their structures, tasks, goals, measures, and coordinating mechanisms place individuals at odds. Such groups are troubled by typical dilemmas: communication failures, struggles for power and influence, unequal or ineffective participation, and decision-making difficulties. Ineffective group processes are often sustained by organizational fictions asserting that particular groups, departments, or units are teams when in reality they are so in name only.

Such fictions exist in caregiving organizations as much as they do elsewhere. The costs may be higher. Real teams enable caregivers to simultaneously join around difficult tasks and provide support to one another. When these teams fail, individuals are left to their own devices. They become their own islands much in the same way that groups split apart from one another to form archipelagos. People turn from one another as potential sources of support. A teaching team meets regularly to review its work with a cohort of students, its members polite but superficial with one another. Members of an executive team of a large residential treatment center maneuver behind the scenes to create political situations favorable to themselves. A surgical team hazes new nurses and technicians, creating disturbing distinctions between senior and junior members. Such teams do not cohere in the face of shared stress and shared tasks. They are marked by internal splits that leave members disconnected from one another.

Boundary integrity

Effective teams are marked by physical, temporal, and psychological boundaries. A surgical team works in an operating room, closed off from the rest of the unit. Its members work together until its operation concludes. Their boundaries are permeable enough to allow members to retrieve information and supplies as necessary, yet impermeable enough to maintain an appropriately sterile environment. Within the operating room they share humor, wear similar uniforms, and weather crises together. When their shift ends, and their operations for the day are complete, the operating room door opens and the team temporarily disbands, its members joining the environment that had been kept at bay while the team worked. The boundaries demarcating the team are dismantled, to appear again when the team needs to reassemble.

Boundaries thus enable team members to turn away from their environments. They keep potentially distracting or noxious stimuli outside. At the same time they bind team members to one another (Smith & Berg 1987). Over time, as doors are closed, meetings held, and joint work effectively performed, team members gradually turn toward one another. They begin to work with and identify with one another. They develop allegiance to their teams. Their team identities occupy more central places in their work lives, shaping what they do and what they think and feel at work. As long as the boundaries around teams are protected, appropriately regulating transactions with their environments, teams may continue to develop into safe places for their members to engage with one another and their tasks.

Teams fail when appropriate boundaries do not exist or are not protected (McCollom 1990). Teams whose members are routinely called out of meetings, assigned to conflicting projects, or given little time to engage in team-related work are simply not strong enough to hold their members. Their members, in turn, are unable to develop allegiances to one another and to shared projects. Similarly, teams that contain members whose primary allegiances are to their particular disciplines, functional areas, departments, or units are marked by internal boundaries that wall members off from one another. Individuals then hold tightly to what might be called *exit relationships*: allegiances and commitments to other groups that permit them, psychologically if not behaviorally, to exit their teams, even as they ostensibly retain their team memberships. Individuals remain committed elsewhere, sliding away from their teams. In doing so, they lay waste to the integrity of boundaries that, like membranes, offer protective layering to healthy organisms.

Fissures

Teams not only exist within but also mirror their contexts. Team members bring with them the issues alive in their organizations. They also import relationships between the organizational and identity groups to which they belong. Rice (1963) has noted that all group processes are intergroup processes. Relations between different functions, departments, disciplines, and organizational status groups, as well as between different racial, gender, age, and ethnic groups, are all routinely enacted within the context of working teams. Just beneath the surface of their work, team members are both re-creating and negotiating the relations between such groupings, which they inescapably represent to one another (Alderfer 1987). Teams are thus micro-cosms: miniature (re)presentations of the intergroup relations marking their organizations. A teaching team is not simply a collection of teachers working on a curriculum. It is also a setting in which individuals representing different disciplinary, seniority, gender, racial, and hierarchical groups re-enact and renegotiate their intergroup relations.

Such groups have their own boundaries relative to one another, which are then imported into the teams themselves. Teams thus exist atop fissures, the fault lines that lie beneath the surface between members representing different groups. When teams encounter stress they cannot withstand it is along such fissures that they crack and split. In caregiving organizations, this stress may be external. It may derive from organizational contexts yet reveal itself in relations among team members. A team of social workers in a social service agency facing mandated downsizing develops tension between its senior and junior members, the latter angry at the likelihood of being let go, the former feeling relieved and guilty. A series of racially motivated student stabbings in a school results in marked conflict between the black and white members of an administrative committee focused on safety issues. A treatment team of residential, educational, and clinical workers charged with reviewing client treatment plans and progress experiences tension between different department members as the organization works to widely imple-ment a controversial new behavior management program. Each of these teams once sought to make its way, steaming toward its given destination. Yet tension within their organizations created waves of pressure that roiled the teams, sending them off course or stopping them altogether.

Stress may also be internal to the team. It may derive from the tasks that members perform, which trigger reactions between team members represent-ing different intergroup affiliations. A team of social workers working with child abuse cases, with little supervision, splits into racial sub-groups, with black and white workers furious at one another for perceived slights and insults. A child cancer unit whose clients have a 50 percent recovery rate becomes the site for a revolt of the nurses against their supervisor, who they experience as insensitive and manipulative. Members of a treatment team working with severely autistic adolescents engage in ongoing fights across disciplinary lines, unable to join together around a shared model of treat-ment. Here too, each of these teams once sought to work well with one another. The stress triggered by their emotionally difficult, seemingly fruitless work, however, exerted a crushing force on their teams. They cracked and split along the underlying intergroup fissures.

In such cases team boundaries either hold or they do not. When they do, team members have drawn together closely enough to create shared responses that help maintain their focus on their team's task. Their team boundary holds; it, and they, prove resilient. When the team boundaries do not hold, team members have drawn away from one another. They employ exit relationships, attaching themselves to their "own" groups. The team's task is lost, along with the integrity of its boundary. Team members are passing ships, on their way to and from the islands on which are beached their "own" groups.

Casualties

This process may create casualties. The team itself might be the casualty. It may be so dysfunctional as to be paralyzed. It may routinely struggle with other parts of the organization, unable to cleanly give and receive information across its boundary. It may be marked by ongoing conflict that never seems to resolve but simply moves around between different actors. Communication is poor. Members are unable to trust one another to act on their behalf. Blame is rife. Work cannot be completed. The team is unable to learn from its mistakes. Old members are replaced by new ones but the dysfunctions persist. Such characteristics are signals that teams themselves have become casualties, crippled by stress of one sort or another.

Teams also have sophisticated, albeit unconscious ways to apportion stress, and in so doing, ensure that only some members become casualties. This enables the team itself to embody some functional aspects, relative to its work, alongside dysfunctional aspects that harm selected members. The basic action is that of splitting and projection. Team members attempt to rid themselves of uncomfortable, unwanted thoughts and feelings by locating them in other team members who unconsciously make themselves available for that purpose (Wells 1985). The process is similar to that described in the previous chapter, in which group members sought to locate unwanted aspects of their selves in members of other groups. Here, the focus is on how this process occurs within teams themselves.

In caregiving organizations in particular, team members become casualties as a result of an often overwhelming, free-floating sense of inadequacy that permeates the system. This experience is endemic, when the needs of careseekers are so large and the resources to serve them so limited. As Mawson (1994) notes, caregivers often seek to dump the anxiety related to their own inadequacy – the sense of not having done enough to save people from pain – into one another rather than reflect together on the idea of the "good enough carer." When they dump on one another a subtle violence is enacted. Individuals are selected to carry some split-off emotion on behalf of the team, while the other parts of their selves are obliterated. A hospital team's anger, pain, and frustration, felt in relation to its work with sick babies, are channeled into its isolation of and fury at the young physician member of the team. Elsewhere a senior nurse is "selected" as the chief "troublemaker," reinforced by other nurses for harassing the physician and ultimately driving her out of the unit (see Obholzer & Roberts 1994). Both the senior nurse and the physician are casualties. Each is reduced to a caricature; each is rendered ineffective to be anything other than what the team wishes her to be.

This process requires all team members to collude. Teams buffeted by external or internal stress seek vulnerable members to contain specific emotions and act out specific issues. This frees up other members to contain other emotions and act out other issues. Together they create a shared defense against the conscious experience of stress and anxiety. Rather than use one another well, in surfacing and confronting that anxiety, they use one another badly: they create casualties of one another, in the form of scapegoats, pariahs, and disgraced leaders. They use one another to rid themselves of painful feelings. Yet those feelings remain within the team, lying in wait to undermine its work.

Sudbury Hospital emergency room

Sudbury Hospital was located in the city of Sudbury, an urban center whose industries had once been strong but had fallen on difficult economic times. The hospital's emergency room (ER) served the city's population, particularly the indigent and the poor who could not afford the services of the suburban hospitals or private physicians. The ER processed an average annual volume of 30,000 patients. It received an average of 25 ambulances each day. The unit contained 17 beds. These were often completely filled, and at times patients were lying in cots stacked against the corridor walls. The ER was obligated to accept all patients, except in the special case when its capacity was so overrun that hospital administrators allowed the unit to temporarily "go on diversion." Ambulance drivers were then instructed to divert all but their sickest patients to other hospital ERs not yet at their capacities. Since hospitals lost money (and valuable patient admissions and surgeries) when their ERs were closed, administrators were often reluctant to go on diversion; when they did so, it was often for no more than a few hours.

Patients visited the Sudbury ER for the full spectrum of reasons, ranging from relatively minor cuts and colds to more critical conditions, including heart attacks, drug overdoses, severed limbs, gunshot wounds, and other medical emergencies. Patients were diagnosed, stabilized and then dealt with in any of several ways: emergency surgeries were transferred to the operating room; serious medical problems were admitted to a hospital unit when a bed became available; chronic diseases, such as alcoholism or psychiatric illness, were referred to other hospital departments for consultation; and minor injuries and complaints were treated and patients discharged. Patients occasionally left without being seen by a physician when the wait became too long. Some were unable to do so given their limited options for medical care.

Both a medical director – a senior ER physician who reported to the hospital president and CEO – and a nurse manager who reported to a vice-president of nursing led the ER department. The ER operated in shifts of teams. Shifts ranged from eight to ten hours. Each team consisted of an ER physician, a physician's assistant, several technicians, and six to eight nurses. The physician on duty was in charge of the medical decisions, while a senior nurse (the charge nurse for the shift) was responsible for deploying the nurses and technicians. The physician's assistant was responsible for a separate room (the "fast track" room) to which the triage nurse guided patients complaining of minor illnesses and injuries. These patients were treated separately, examined more cursorily by the attending physician, and usually discharged quickly.

I conducted an organizational diagnosis of the Sudbury ER, which occurred over the course of several months of observations and interviews, and culminated in a series of feedback meetings with department members. The themes presented below were part of the feedback material.

The caged

The ER staff dealt with patients in distress. The patients were sick, often frightened, and presented ambiguous complaints and incomplete information. Many had no other place to go, and wished for the ER staff to quickly relieve their pain. They presented all this – their fear, their dependency, and their anxiety – to the ER staff. The ER was routinely understaffed, owing to the generally precarious financial nature of the hospital itself as well as to the lack of trained ER physicians and nurses in the region. This was particularly acute for the nurses, who regularly worked overtime. Short-handed, they also had to cover more patients in less time. Team members were often anxious about compromising patient care because of understaffing.

A patient population whose illnesses had historically been treated in psychiatric facilities and various shelters also heightened the stress. With the closing of those institutions, the patients sought free care and shelter in the ER. These patients were often abusive. This was distracting for the staff, taking attention away from truly medical issues and emergencies. It was also frightening. Without police or security personnel to protect them or calm the patients, ER staff members were fearful, often with good reason, of assaults by disturbed or disruptive patients. These patients remained in the ER for many hours when there was no other place for them to go or because of long waits for consultations from the psychiatric or detoxification units. ER staff referred to their unit as the "dumping ground" for the city's indigent population.

The ER staff's primary experience was frustration, routinely expressed towards one another, patients, hospital administrators and other units, and grounded in their inability to control their boundaries. Ambulances arrived unpredictably. Patients walked in off the street. Except when the ER was clearly overwhelmed and went on diversion, the unit was unable to turn people away. They also had little control over the flow of patients out of the unit. While they could discharge patients they treated for relatively minor problems, they could not easily admit more seriously ill patients without the involvement and permission of physicians and nurses in other units. Nor could they control the timing of consultations from other hospital services, which were often understaffed as well. The charge nurse, ostensibly in charge of monitoring patient flow, was often pressed into duty as a nurse to cover for the understaffing of many shifts. The unit then overflowed with patients, their beds jamming the hallways.

The ER staff was thus left to contain the patients. The patients themselves grew increasingly frustrated as their waiting times lengthened. They often directed their anger at the ER staff. Some did this relatively gently while others lost control, made helpless by fear, longing, drunkenness, or mental illness. Since there were no separate areas for psychiatric patients, their anxiety was funneled into the rest of the unit, stirring up the emotions of other patients and staff alike. The waiting room outside the unit, filled with family members and patients waiting to be admitted, held more anxiety. The opening of the door to the ER, as a nurse came out to collect patients, was greeted by waiting room members with hope (that the door would deliver them from uncertainty and anxiety), disappointment (when the call was for another), and anger (that they had to remain in their agitated state). ER staff members did not much like to cross the boundary into the waiting room, wishing to keep others' anxiety at bay.

The ER staff thus felt jammed. They were unable to move the flow of patients more quickly. Their borders were under attack: one doorway was for ambulances; the other led to the waiting area. The physical layout of the ER offered little respite. The main room contained eight beds. Only flimsy curtains drawn around the beds separated the patients. The ER staff needed to monitor the patients constantly and were thus themselves constantly on display. There were no back office areas to which they could retreat, save a worn changing room containing lockers, a table, and several chairs. They lacked what Goffman (1959) refers to as a "backstage" area where they could safely decompress from their "on-stage" experiences. The ER staff were caged: on display, unable to leave, dealing with a series of often stressful tasks from which there was no physical escape. As the flow of patients out of the unit slowed, pressure mounted with little hope of appropriate release.

Retreats, full and partial

ER members created various strategies for coping with the chronic frustration related to their inability to control the boundaries of their unit. Some strategies enabled members to perform their tasks quite well. This was particularly true for the weekday night shift, whose members shared their frustrations with one another, helped one another with difficult patients, and regularly asked for and received help during their shift. Other strategies, practiced by most of the other shift teams, were self-protective and did little to aid the work itself. Individual staff members, unable to manage their physical space and protect their unit's boundaries, psychologically distanced themselves and protected their personal boundaries. This is not uncommon in hospitals, where staff members unconsciously fear attachments and dependency on colleagues and superiors, as if such connections would trigger emotional demands that threaten competence (Dartington 1994).

This played out differently across the ER's disciplines. The nurses and technicians husbanded their resources in order to protect their energies. In the extreme, they stayed home, taking sick or personal days. Such "call-ins" increased the amount of work on other team members, creating more stress and frustration for the unit to bear. More routinely, they created cliques within the teams. Small groups of nurses or technicians sat and socialized while other team members worked. These splits were enabled by the informal assigning of nurses to specific patients (according to rooms) whom they defined as "their own"; unless it was a life-threatening emergency, they rarely extended themselves to help with other nurses' patients. They also distanced themselves from one another in their communications. They could be short-tempered with one another, and at times were plainly disrespectful and rude. They blamed rather than sought to understand one another and this created inappropriate boundaries that kept each party at bay.

The nurses and technicians also sought to keep patients at some remove. The physical layout of the ER did not allow for private conversations among staff members. Staff responded by acting as if the patients were not there. They spoke openly to one another in the course of their work, not only about their work tasks but also about the patients themselves – their present-ing problems, their dispositions, their physical characteristics. Such lack of professionalism was motivated by anger at the non-medical patients (i.e., alcoholics, drug abusers, psychiatric patients) who were not likely to use their care in the unit to interrupt their diseases. This frustrated the staff. As Dartington (1994) notes, nurses need "good enough" patients who need nurses and get better with their care. The ER's patients deprived the staff of the opportunity to receive gratification and feel deeply satisfied. The staff distanced themselves from patients who were unable to provide such satisfaction.

The physicians also distanced themselves from both staff and patients. Many retreated into the role of expert. Their interactions with both staff and patients had the quality and pacing of the hit-and-run: the physician would enter a room, scan the chart, examine the patient, instruct the nurse, and then move on, hurrying to the next patient, and not incidentally, reducing personal involvements with staff and patients alike. They were disinclined to share information with or listen respectfully to nurses and technicians. The physicians distanced themselves from hospital administrators as well, blaming them for the understaffing, the removal of police from the unit, and their refusals to go on diversion. The physician group was thus an island unto itself; its members moved alone through their shifts, dispensing orders and prescriptions for staff and patients to follow.

Teams divided

These strategies reduced teamwork during many of the shifts. Nurses identified with and attached themselves to particular assignments, tasks, patients, and co-workers. They disassociated themselves from the team as a whole. The technicians, as the low-status group, interacted primarily with one another. The physicians moved quickly among everyone, darting here and there. Communication across these actors was sparse, incomplete, often disjointed. Or it was noisy, filled with the static of frustration, anger, and negativity with which staff members regarded their situations, their patients, and in particular, one another, from whom they had walled themselves off by means of the psychological boundaries they constructed. These boundaries also had physical manifestations. The ER could be mapped as a collection of rooms with little traffic between them: the fast track room, the triage desk, the nurses' station, patient rooms, the physician's desk. Staff members strayed into but rarely remained in others' territory.

The teams split along certain disciplinary fissures, particularly that of physicians and nurses. Physicians often left little room for the nurses to do real nursing – to engage their own faculties and intuitions in making sense of the patients' complaints and arrive at a preliminary diagnosis to present to the attending physician, to be a partner in implementing, if not developing, the treatment plan. Nurses often ended up surprised by the treatment plans, leaving them both less effective at, and more dissatisfied with, the implementation process. Nurses dealt with such seeming arrogance by choosing when and how to follow the physician's instructions. Physicians had little formal control over the nurses, who were accountable to their own manager. The physicians were thus at the mercy of the nurses, and often had to ask nurses to perform tasks "as a favor." In place of teamwork, then, there was an economy of personal relationships between physicians and nurses, who often made decisions according to their personal histories with one another.

Within the nursing group, there were divisions between senior and junior nurses. Those who had been with the hospital for some time tended to join together during their shifts, socializing while the more junior nurses worked their rooms. The relatively new nurses – both permanent, younger nurses and the temporary, *per diem* nurses – were left to fend for themselves. Some were fortunate and enlisted a mentor. The others colluded with the prevailing norms, forming cliques with like-minded nurses or withdrawing from others altogether. These distinctions fell away, however, as the nurses drew sharper distinctions between themselves and the technicians, refusing (or with great resentment and under duress agreeing) to perform some of the tasks – transporting patients, cleaning rooms, replenishing supplies – they considered inappropriate to their level of expertise.

The divisions within the teams directly impacted on the staff's ability to care for the patients. Decisions were made about when and how to care for patients according to whether staff members liked or were angry at one another. Patients were left in need despite the availability of nurses who did not wish to help others with "their" patients. Information about patients' conditions was not provided or not heeded because of staff members' artless disrespect of one another. Treatment plans were not shared, making it difficult to order laboratory tests, plan patient transitions to other units, and the like. The sketchy communication within teams made it difficult to examine practices and develop consistent protocols. Such splits within the teams inevitably shaped their abilities to turn together to meet the needs of their patients in appropriate, timely ways.

Self-perpetuating cycles

These divisions were held in place by self-perpetuating cycles. These cycles were variations on a theme: team members distanced themselves from one another, which created more stress and tension, fueled individuals' desires for self-protection, and led to increased distancing from one another. These cycles continued, uninterrupted, to the point where they defined the culture of most of the unit's teams.

There were four variations on this theme within the unit. Two occurred within the nursing group. First, when nurses did not help one another during their shifts, workload inequities were created: some nurses worked hard, others did not. Those who worked hard became stressed and resentful. They then distanced themselves from the others; they became like them, slacking off and not helping others in order not to be unfairly burdened. Second, when the more experienced, senior nurses did not support or teach the less experienced, junior nurses, the latter were unable to work efficiently enough to help reduce the load on the team more generally. The senior nurses grew resentful. They then withdrew from the junior nurses, who withdrew from others or left altogether, causing still more stress for the remaining team members.

The third variation revolved around the ER members' shared frustration with their lack of control over the forces that threatened to overwhelm them daily: the staffing issues, patient flow through and out of the unit, the unpredictability of patient arrivals, and the nature of the patient population itself. Members acted out their frustration against one another, treating colleagues disrespectfully, rudely, and unprofessionally. This undermined their trust in and respect for one another, which in turn detracted from their ability to turn toward one another for support. Unable to join together and draw upon one another's resources – and thus unable to create a unified approach to the forces acting upon them – they experienced less control over their environment than they otherwise might, and this maintained their frustration.

The fourth variation involved the unit's relationships with other hospital units. The charge nurses were responsible for working with their counterparts in other units to determine the appropriate places to admit patients. The ER staff resented other units for their perceived non-responsiveness to the need to relieve the pressure on the ER. This resentment was channeled into the ER charge nurses, who acted out against other units' representatives. Communication was worsened between the ER and other units, whose representatives grew frustrated with the ER and moved to process its requests more slowly. This in turn heightened the frustration within the ER staff, whose members felt confirmed in their perceptions of other units as non-responsive.

Casting calls

These cycles may be understood as social defenses, held in place because they shielded members from examining and confronting their powerlessness, rage, fears, and anxieties about their performance. In order to maintain these defenses the teams required individual staff members to perform particular roles. Individuals needed to be the objects of others' projections and to act in ways that guaranteed that those projections would continue. Specific members thus auditioned for and were cast in certain roles.

The narcissistic leader

The medical director of the ER was widely perceived as self-absorbed, narcissistic, and concerned primarily with protecting the physicians rather than the ER and the integrity of its teams. He was liked but not trusted. Staff members, including some physicians, acknowledged that the medical director spoke "doublespeak," thoughtlessly making vague and conflicting promises to different people. He was, in the words of one staff member, "like smoke": unsubstantial, wispy. He was ineffective at protecting the unit's boundaries. The hospital administration did not trust him, based on his inciting the unit against them, and he isolated himself and the unit from other hospital units. He modeled the lack of personal responsibility for the unit. His role enabled the unit to cast blame elsewhere – on him, on the administrators – and relieved members of the responsibility of examining their own culpability in how they worked with one another.

The troublemaker

A male nurse, a leading representative of the powerful nursing union, was cast in the role of chief troublemaker. He was constantly agitating for more staff, money, benefits, and other resources for the nurses. His reputation with the other nurses on his team was poor: he was perceived as a slacker and a consistent source of negativity, pointing out contractual issues that divided team members according to different unions. Still, others would complain to him about understaffing, missed lunches, overtime and the like. This kept him in a relatively permanent state of rage toward the administration and its representatives, which he expressed on behalf of other unit members. While many of the issues that he raised had merit, his adversarial stance kept them from serious consideration on the part of the administration, which sought to fire him.

The abuser

A senior female nurse, on the hospital staff for 30 years, contained and expressed the unit's mounting anger toward the patient population. The nurse had a reputation for brusqueness toward the patients but had become increasingly rude and dismissive, addressing them as "drunks" and "psychos." Other team members had tolerated this, in that the behavior was allowed to continue with few consequences. It was at the point when she crossed a normative boundary and pushed a patient that the administration moved against her, temporarily suspending her. Also suspended was the unit's ability to express its collective, unspoken rage against the patients, both for their abusiveness and their inabilities to let the nurses save them.

The victim

A technician specializing in orthopedics and assigned to assist an orthopedic surgeon set bones and apply splints worked in a room devoted to that purpose. Over a period of several months she was anonymously harassed by a group of nurses working other shifts. They left threatening notes and defaced pictures and other personal property she left in the orthopedic room. Other staff members were aware of these violations but did little to halt them. The technician thus became the repository of a set of interrelated emotions: violation, fear, vulnerability, anger, and helplessness. She contained those emotions on behalf of others, who felt similarly in relation to the violation of the unit's boundaries by the patients. The technician became the symbolic victim for the team, taking as her own the victimization of all staff members. Her selection was inspired both by her low-status position as a technician and her location in a separate room with boundaries that could be violated.

Ms Incompetent

A young nurse hired after only recently completing her training worked on a team in the unit. She was not paired with any senior members of the team but was thrown into the work. She was, for the most part, left alone. She worked slowly. It took her longer to locate supplies, perform procedures with patients, finish paperwork, and complete her other tasks. She made mistakes, which the physicians would bring to her attention, some more gently than others. The other nurses on her shift largely abandoned her; instead, they socialized with one another, laughingly making predictions about how long new nurses would last in the unit. They thus sought to locate within her the sense of incompetence and failure that they, as a team, felt in relation to their work with patients, and the sense of loneliness and abandonment they felt in relation to one another and the hospital more generally. The team let this occur, moved by the unconscious wish to have her, rather than they, feel and contain those emotions.

Dr Fragility

The only female physician was perceived as excessively fragile, prone to anx-iety, a producer of heightened emotion rather than calm in the unit. Her boundaries were weak, as she confided inappropriately in nurses and bent the rules with patients. She also established relatively close relationships with staff, and grew attached to some patients. The nurses and technicians sought to take care of her in various ways: calming her down when she grew upset by some logistical problem, withholding information that they knew would upset her, and taking care of some issues themselves rather than make demands upon her. They also liked her, and socialized with her in ways they did not with the other physicians. They appreciated her focus on relationships with them and with her patients, which flew in the face of team members' strategies of distance and detachment. She was punished for this by being perceived and treated as weak and fragile.

The abandoned

The physician's assistant worked largely alone in the fast track area, located down a long corridor of the ER. He treated a small segment of the patients, with whom other team members rarely interacted because of their relatively minor ailments. The assistant was left for long stretches of time without nursing or physician support: no nurses or technicians were assigned to that room, and the physicians were often too busy caring for the other patients to do more than sign the paperwork the assistant prepared for patient discharges. The assistant felt cloistered and lonely. On behalf of the unit, he contained the sense of abandonment that other team members experienced in relation to the hospital and its surrounding community. The fast track area became the "dumping ground" for patients, a smaller version of how the ER itself was the dumping ground for the community more generally, who deposited its indigent and sick on its doors and backed away. The ER located and sealed off the resulting feelings – of frustration, anger, abandonment, longing – within the physician's assistant.

The savior

The new nurse manager was widely perceived as a calming presence in the unit. She was clear-eyed, insightful and trustworthy in her communications and interactions with unit members. Personally hired by the hospital's vice-president of nursing, she was perceived as having influence with senior administrators. She focused her early efforts on issues of accountability, equity, teamwork, and creating a culture of respect rather than blame and negativity. She earned respect from her nurses, and later the technicians and physicians. She was cast as the teller of truth and substance, the antidote to the wispy narcissism of the medical director. Over time she became identified with team members' stirrings of hope and change. They referred to her as the fixer, the one who would make things in the unit right. In doing so they located the responsible parts of themselves within her, as if she would save them rather than help them save themselves from their dysfunctional patterns. She would nurse them to health, and they would wait for her medicine to work.

These roles served functions so important in the unconscious life of the ER teams that their occupants were sacrificed. Individuals became uni-dimensional. They were perceived as if they were only that which they appeared to others – as fragile, narcissistic, incompetent, abusive, or victimized. They each colluded with this as well. This allowed them identities that felt acceptable, if not familiar or necessary, according to their own personal histories. They also served their teams, in the way of soldiers falling on grenades as they explode, saving others as they destroyed themselves. In the ER, however, the truth was more complicated and people were less heroic and selfless, as ostensible team-mates covertly pushed vulnerable others toward falling grenades. They did so in the service of their unit's social defenses.

Team defenses

The ER teams' social defenses defended the whole at the expense of some of its parts. The sacrificed parts were individual team members cast into roles that required them to contain certain emotions on behalf of the others. "Dr Fragility" contained weakness. "Ms Incompetent" contained ineffectualness. "The abuser" contained rage. "The abandoned" contained isolation and rejection. Such emotions were rife within the team more generally. The experience of the ER unit, in relation to its work with its patients, was that it was ineffectual and weak (from being unable to heal or fix chronically ill patients, or manage its own boundaries), enraged (from being assigned an impossible task), and isolated and rejected (by the hospital and the community more generally). The experience also involved satisfaction and joy in saving others' lives, and a moral clarity that the work itself was meaningful and true.

Rather than have all unit members experience these difficult, often contradictory emotions, the ER teams unconsciously colluded to simplify their experiences. They untangled the emotions from one another and parceled them out to specific individuals. Through splitting and projection, individuals became identified with specific emotions. This enabled others to not have to experience them so profoundly. As long as "the abandoned" felt rejected and isolated, other team members could feel joined to and nurtured by one another. As long as "Ms Incompetent" felt unsure and ineffectual, other team members felt sure and competent. As long as "the victim" felt harassed and frightened, other team members felt safer and fearless. The ER teams needed these individuals to feel these emotions such that others would not have to. The teams were staging plays whose plots invariably involved treating some members in particular ways – such as isolating them, feeding their rage, or refusing to help them – that would continuously fill them with the emotions they were assigned to carry.

The assigned individuals colluded with this partly because it served unconscious needs for them. The emotions they carried may have felt familiar or satisfied some need they had. Yet some of them also had few options. The ER unit projected difficult emotions onto individuals who had relatively little power to reject them. "Ms Incompetent" was a junior nurse, with little seniority. "The victim" was a technician, the lowest-status group in the unit. "Dr Fragility" was the only female physician. "The troublemaker" was relatively unskilled as a nurse. "The narcissistic leader" was gay and Hispanic, and marginalized by hospital administrators. These characteristics made it difficult for these people to reject the roles into which they were cast. They were provided niches in the ER, which offered them a sort of power that they otherwise lacked. Their power was located less in their ability to change their circumstances than in their ability to contain difficult emotions for others. They were given bit parts by the core of the ER – the senior nurses, the male physicians – who were left relatively protected from difficult emotional experiences.

At play here were parallel processes. The relationship between the relatively powerless individuals and the relatively powerful core of the ER teams paralleled that between the ER and the hospital more generally. The unit contained a difficult patient population, which was admitted slowly, if at all, into other parts of the hospital. The patients – and the frustration, rage, impotence, incompetence, and victimization they triggered in others – were thus split off from the rest of the hospital and contained in the ER. The ER was forced to keep those patients. It kept within its boundaries the emotions triggered by the work with these patients, given that there was no other place

– not the administration, not the community, not the other units of the hospital – in which those emotions could be released. So the unit found individuals into which, like vessels, they could pour those emotions. There were other parallel processes as well. The inequity issues among the nurses paralleled the relationship between the ER and other hospital units. The intensive care unit and other hospital units were not pitching in to relieve some of the burden of the ER unit by admitting their patients. The hospital thus treated the unit in ways that were unconsciously picked up and re-enacted among ER members.

The ER's defenses remained uninterrupted, as teams were unable to reflect on their own processes. They had no forums in which to examine how they acted out their collective frustration, anger, abandonment, and powerlessness in their own relations. When tensions rose – patients were spilling out of rooms and lying in the corridors, were disruptive and abusive, or could not be admitted to other units – team members withdrew from one another. Their contacts became sharper, less forgiving. They withdrew into isolated pockets of relationships and treated one another disrespectfully. They abandoned one another. Precisely when ER teams needed to coalesce, their members drawing together to figure out how to gain control over their seemingly hopeless situation, the teams fell back on defenses that ensured that such connections could not occur.

From scarcity to safety

Felt scarcity – of attention, honor, love – is the fundamental disturbance in group life (Gustafson & Cooper 1985). In the ER teams, members experienced scarcity keenly. There was scarcity of attention, from the community and the hospital. Scarce also was the nurturing, valuing, and respecting of team members, who felt themselves under assault from the patient population. The teams became disturbed. The hospital sustained the fiction that the ER teams were real but in practice they were not. Members could not join together on the shared task of caring for all patients together. Instead, they split apart along various fissures – discipline, seniority, gender – and sought to locate the pain of the scarcity within one another.

It does not have to be this way, of course. Teams in caregiving organizations often get loaded up with various dynamics that swirl within the organizations themselves. They are microcosms: smaller, easily digestible representations of dynamics at play in their embedding systems. Team members are drawn to acting out the relations between their teams and their organization. Members *use* one another as their teams are used by their organizations; ER teams were abandoned rather than joined with and absorbed by the hospital, leading to team members being abandoned rather than absorbed by one another. Such parallel processes offer the very real opportunity for learning. Team members can examine their team dynamics for valuable lessons about organizational dynamics. Indeed, one reason why organizations create and maintain ineffective teams is that they are unconsciously seeking help in interrupting the dysfunctional patterns in which their members are caught. They do so by offering a more easily understood forum – teams – for examination.

Such covert "communications" work if teams are able to interrupt their own re-enactments of the dysfunctional patterns. If they cannot, they will continue to be used to serve organizational social defenses. They will continue as casualties of those defenses, with the most acute pain and disturbance located within the most vulnerable team members. Interrupting such patterns requires team members to confront the paradox of safety (Smith & Berg 1987): members must act as if it is safe enough to speak freely of their experiences, even when they feel it is not, given the splits they have created. Leaders must act as if the creation of such safety is of paramount concern, and make it so.

Certain organizational structures and processes can aid the creation of safety. As noted in the previous chapter, caregiving organization units, such as teams, need to function within boundaries that press members to turn towards rather than away from one another. Regular team meetings that begin and end on time, with clear agendas and tasks, and a focus on raising and solving problems, help create such boundaries. So does the practice of confidentiality. At the core of creating safety, however, are the ways that members engage one another. Over time, and with the right facilitation or consultation, group members can learn to disclose increasingly authentic parts of themselves – what they really think and feel about their work experiences and one another. Together, they can examine those thoughts and feelings for the clues or information that they may contain about careseekers' experiences or their own social defenses. If they are able to act as if such conversations are possible, they become so.

In the final analysis, caregiving organization teams are functional to the extent that their members look to one another to share the burden of careseekers' distress. In dysfunctional teams, the true scarcity is members' attentiveness to one another. They cast one another into roles that wall them off from one another. They seek exit relationships that leave them held, in some fashion, and leave their purported team-mates to make their own ways. Reversing this dynamic requires acts of leadership, and of "followership." Leaders, formal or informal, need to emerge and push themselves and their teams toward sustained examinations of how and why they function as they do, and the consequences for their abilities to work and to manage stress. Team members need to follow, acting as if it is safe to speak honestly when, at some level of awareness, they know it is not. Such concerted movements toward anxiety – in the context of regular team meetings devoted both to problems and processes – are the building blocks of resilience for teams, their members, and ultimately, caregiving organizations themselves.

Chapter 9

Politics

Politics in caregiving organizations is much like what occurs elsewhere. Individuals strive for power, position and prestige. They align with influential others to move ahead their projects and interests. They join with others in formal groups or informal coalitions. They seek to acquire, enhance and use power and other resources to obtain their preferred outcomes. Such activities may be quite rational. They can define a process by which scarce resources are allocated to people and ideas that gain enough influence and constituents to emerge as acceptable paths through ambiguity and uncertainty. Political behavior is then a process by which organization members vet possible directions; those ultimately selected are those that serve the interests of the most (or the most important) constituencies.

Politics in organizations is thus distantly related to democratic politics. Both operate on the principle that the competing interests of various groups and constituencies will vie in various forums, out of which will emerge solutions that garner enough resources and power to influence the larger system. Both hold to the notion that the rightness of ideas about how best to achieve preferred outcomes shall emerge through a process by which proponents seek to persuade others, gaining champions and momentum. In practice, of course, this process can be corrupted. Individuals and organizations may wield undue influence based not on the power of ideas and solutions but on that of relationships, unfair practices, or coercion that build alliances and coalitions and generate commitments that serve their own interests more so than those of their organizations. It is through such practices that organizational politics, often a useful tool by which organizations identify appropriate strategy and necessary changes, comes to be viewed with skepticism.

Organizational permeability

Politics in caregiving organizations are further complicated by relatively permeable boundaries in relation to their environments. Caregiving work requires that careseekers have relatively unfettered access to caregivers.

Hospital doors swing open to admit patients rushing to emergency rooms or appearing for laboratory tests, physician exams, or medical procedures. Schools serve their communities, enrolling students from surrounding neighborhoods. Churches and synagogues welcome worshippers to their services and members to their congregations. Treatment centers accept clients as long as they have the relevant disorders or problems, have access to insurance or private funds, and are likely to improve through treatment. Shelters take in the homeless or indigent who have no other place to go. Careseekers thus stream into caregiving organizations with relatively few restrictions on their entry.

Careseekers bring with them the multitude of issues, divisions, contradictions, and wishes contained in the larger society. Each type of caregiving organization exists at a societal intersection of ambivalence, competing theories and ideals, and anxiety. In the first chapter I described how careseekers are brought into and "digested" by caregiving organizations, inevitably importing into those organizations the societal issues and struggles attached to caregiving tasks. Residential institutions struggle with conflicts around "warehousing" or "growing" clients. Schools struggle with conflicts between developing the creative, critical faculties of individuals and ensuring the standardized equality of all students. Hospitals struggle with tensions between patient care and educating physicians, conducting funded research, and ensuring profits. These tensions exist within society, which is genuinely torn between different ideals and goals.

Such tensions shape how individual careseekers are "digested" and provided for. They are also reproduced in caregiving organizations more generally, given that many caregiving organizations are "underbounded," i.e., they have more boundary permeability than is optimal. They risk becoming overwhelmed by environmental turbulence to the point that they lose a consistent sense of their own identity (Alderfer 1980a). When organizations have strong boundaries and a clear sense of their mission and goals, everyday turbulence has little lasting effect, like air currents that temporarily shake a passing airplane. When organizations have weak boundaries and a conflicted sense of their missions and goals, they do not simply pass through turbulence, the turbulence infiltrates the organization. Societal tensions about how to best educate next generations of children, care for emotionally abused adolescents in residential settings, and care for the elderly, to name a few, leak into school buildings, treatment centers, and nursing homes. These organizations become microcosms of the societies in which they are embedded.

Political behavior in caregiving organizations, then, is often in reality struggles between different ideologies, approaches, interests, and groups in society more generally. These struggles are imported into caregiving organizations and waged just beneath the surface of overt struggles for resources, influence, direction, and other vital elements of organizational life.

Organization members are not simply vying for their own personal interests, nor are organizational groups simply trying to protect their own turf. Rather, they are acting out, in ways often unbeknownst to them, larger societal conflicts. A residential treatment center has a simmering conflict between administrators who want the clients more controlled and caseworkers who want the clients more autonomous. A public high school's teachers are split between those who support and those who decry standardized testing. A hospital contains ongoing battles between researchers and primary care physicians competing for space and resources. Each of these struggles represents a larger split in society. They are imported into the caregiving organizations, in the unconscious hope that they will be resolved there.

Politics in caregiving organizations thus play out at multiple levels simultaneously. At one level there are organizational politics as they are typically enacted and driven by individuals, groups, and cultures in organizational life. At another level there are societal splits, ambiguities, and tensions around the primary tasks of caregiving organizations that are imported into those organizations. Organizations become the available arenas for the working out of societal issues. Individuals and groups take up different parts of the issues and try and solve them on behalf of the larger society in which they function. The means of resolution may vary greatly. Organization members may frame projects that call for a reasoned resolution of different approaches. Leaders may define organizational tasks in ways that embrace one approach and suppress others. Members may sort themselves into different factions and wage conflict, sending forth leaders like gladiators to do battle. Each of these represents an attempt to manage the environmental turbulence that infiltrates a caregiving organization.

Social anxiety

Caregiving organization members' attempts to resolve the various tensions, splits, and ambiguities associated with primary tasks are made difficult by the anxiety those tasks trigger within the larger society. The task of education, for example, raises a general anxiety about the survival of the next generation. Children and other learners need to be taught the tools they need to survive. Such responsibility is relegated to communities, schools, and teachers, onto which parents project their fears about their own children's survival, sense of inadequacy, and hopes for what cannot easily occur – namely, that all children will be equally well-equipped to meet all of life's challenges (Obholzer 1994). Consider, as a small instance, a parent's terror that her child is being left behind in some fundamental way. The child is not learning as quickly, making friends as easily, or adapting as smoothly as other children. The parent's anxiety, which may present itself as anger, sadness, guilt, shame, or any combination thereof, is brought into the school through interactions with the child's teacher and other school personnel. Multiply this by a hundredfold for a glimpse of the anxiety that routinely permeates the boundaries of any school.

Similarly, the tasks of healthcare and ministry raise social anxiety about death and dying and the meaning, of life. People take their wishes for immortality and freedom from pain, their terrors of death and its annihilation of all they have known, and their longings for certainty and meaning, and project them onto hospitals and religious institutions. Such social anxiety is the backdrop upon which caregiving organizations exist. It is omnipresent, constantly imported into organizations by careseekers. Consider a mother's incoherent rage and grief as her child struggles with a painful, wracking disease; a man's mounting frustration and sadness as his lover seems to get better and then suddenly worsens; a woman battling a mental illness that does not yield to psychiatric ministrations or drugs, and whose spiritual practices at church offer little relief. Multiply a hundredfold as well, for a sense of the layers of anxiety that pervade these institutions.

Caregiving organizations thus contain anxieties for society as a whole. They are the places upon which people more generally project their needs, hopes, fears, and anxieties about survival, pain, death, and other forms of loss and annihilation. Caregiving organization members have their own anxieties as well, triggered both by their personal experiences in the role of careseekers and their contacts with others' anxieties. They inevitably create shared defenses against anxiety that, as described previously, distract organization members from the underlying sources of their anxiety. Members thus alter their primary tasks in order to reduce the pain associated with their direct engagement (Obholzer 1994).

Social defenses may derive form and power from the larger society flooding through caregiving organizations. Political behavior in these organizations is intimately related to social defenses. It is driven by what Shapiro and Carr (1991: 169) describe as "the simplest and more obvious group defense . . . which is to generate a series of polarities: subgroups are identified and members join them in order to establish some form of identity."

Sub-groups become the focus for stereotyped projections. This enables organization members to substitute the tasks of vying for resources, ideas, influence, and supremacy between groups for those focused on careseekers' needs. Sub-groups, which are on the surface at odds with one another are, beneath the surface, colluding with one another to distract organization members from social anxiety.

The polarities by which political behavior is enacted within caregiving organizations mirror the larger society. Primary conflicts are played out through identity groups (Alderfer 1980a). These are affiliations that help individuals shape their personal identities, including generation groups (e.g., young, middle-aged), gender groups (men and women), racial groups (e.g., African-American, Caucasian), religious groups (e.g., Muslim, Christian, Jewish), and ethnic groups (e.g., English, African, Irish). Individuals inevitably represent these groups in their interactions with one another, to the point that interpersonal relationships may be understood as intergroup relationships. In underbounded systems, conflicts between identity groups, imported from the surrounding environment, tend to supplant those between work groups (Alderfer 1980a). The politicized sub-groups in caregiving organizations that are particularly susceptible to their environments, like public schools and community hospitals, are likely to be those that exist within the society at large.

This adds a complicated layering to the nature of social defenses. The politics of race, gender, and ethnicity, to name a few, leak through porous organization boundaries and shape defenses against anxiety. Often enough, this overwhelms efforts to move past such defenses. "In the contemporary world," note Shapiro and Carr (1991: 169), "such divisions of race and gender evoke familiar and strong feelings. Any effort to explore the underlying dynamics behind the pressured need to create such stereotyped groups is often washed away in floods of socially legitimate, and therefore unquestioned and uninterpreted, pronouncements." Society uses rhetoric and stereotypes to simplify complicated issues – of equality, justice, responsibility, and opportunity – and render them unsolvable. Caregiving organizations mimic this process.

In this chapter I present an analysis of the politics surrounding the implementation of a new program in an urban public high school. The analysis focuses on the irrational as well as rational purposes of organizational politics – that is, on their defensive as well as expressive dimensions. The case study draws heavily upon action research within urban high schools conducted by Michelle Fine (1994), Linda Powell (1994, 1997), Nancy Zane (1994), and their colleagues.

Thurston High School

Thurston High School served an American urban area blighted by drugs, crime, and poverty. The surrounding neighborhoods were marked by boarded-up row houses, empty storefronts, and loitering men. Of the 2000 students in the school, 80 percent were on some form of public assistance. They represented a mixed population of the urban poor, heavily dominated by racial minorities and immigrants, with a minority of white students. Bars covered the windows of the school. The walls were sprayed with a cacophony of paint and slogans. Guards armed with guns and walkie-talkies patrolled the halls, alert for the violence that occasionally erupted between students representing neighborhood gangs. Students and teachers alike attempted to work amidst a climate of fear and hopelessness.

Students organized themselves into warring cliques. Their teachers changed every year and rarely formed ongoing relationships with individual students. Many students were anonymous within Thurston, the exceptions being those who managed to stand out through behavioral problems or, more rarely, academic excellence. This paralleled teachers' relations with one another. Thurston's teachers had a great deal of autonomy within their classrooms, which in practice translated into isolation from one another. They spent little time talking with one another about teaching practices, they had few personal connections, and their own relations paralleled the distance and anonymity of their relations with the students.

The teachers' disconnection was not simply a matter of the size of the school or amount of work they had to do. It represented a set of individual and social defenses against the anxiety triggered by the task of working with the population of students (Powell 1994). As Kozol (1991) describes, few adults are prepared to confront the daily ravages of hunger, hopelessness, family stress, and political powerlessness. Most turn away, toward defense mechanisms enabling them to live and work in denial. As long as the teachers had little connection to the students, and knew little about their personal lives, they did not have to experience difficult feelings. They did not have to take in and digest the pain, anger and sadness that the students – who lived with poverty, abuse, homelessness, drugs, teen pregnancy and abortion, suicide – represented.

The teachers' social defense was to remain disconnected from their students. They knew their students as little more than a series of English essays or mathematics scores. They taught their classes, engaged with students around academic content when they were not disciplining them, and sought relief in the teachers' lounge. They resisted students' attempts to draw them closer, to engage with them as individuals with particular hopes, experiences, and difficulties. Fine (1994: 26) describes this defense as relatively routine:

> There are good reasons that faculty become burned out or callous to students' lives. Educators today are picking up the pieces of a society ravaged by class and race stratification, and they are being held account-able for transforming students who carry the weight of the bottom of the social hierarchy into educated and optimistic citizens. In particular, high school educators have inherited histories of academic defeat, that they need to reverse. In this process, many educators, though certainly not all, have opted not to know the pains and struggles experienced by their students. "If I knew," said one very committed teacher, "what would I do?"

Maintaining one's distance from students was thus a way for teachers to not feel hopeless, angry, sad, guilty, and, finally, impotent in the face of seemingly overwhelming odds against their students escaping the "bottom." They chose loneliness and isolation over attaching to others in pain.

Such choices held certain implications for the school. Students, left without secure attachments to adults at school, responded in various ways. Some simply disengaged, withdrawing temporarily (attendance at Thurston hovered around 65 percent) or permanently (the dropout rate was 25 percent). Others showed little interest in learning; standardized scores remained far below the national mean. Still others were enraged, often without quite knowing why. They erupted in violence, mostly against other students, occasionally toward teachers. They were disrespectful with one another and with the teachers and administrator, who, it seemed, had given up on them.

Battling for control

Thurston was often preoccupied with disciplinary issues. Teachers felt locked in a battle with students for control of the school (see Zane 1994). The teachers represented themselves as the passive victims of students' disruptive behavior, blaming students individually ("the bad apples") or generally ("the breed of students"). They recognized that many of the students were in difficult familial situations, contributing to high absenteeism and poor grades, and in response lowered their expectations. In place of emphasizing academic excellence they focused on discipline. "Good classes" were defined less in terms of students' engagement with academic material than in terms of less problem students disrupting classes. The school focused on establishing disciplinary codes to hold students accountable.

Such battles for discipline and control are usually held in place by teachers and administrators blaming students and their parents (Zane 1994). At Thurston, students who acted out – by skipping school, dropping out, becoming physically or verbally abusive, disrupting classes – were considered to have personal problems which could be controlled through clear, systemic standards and rules. The teachers disparaged the students' parents for their seeming inability to control their children or spark their academic interest. The parents were neither welcomed nor integrated into the school. This reinforced their distance from their children's education, which enabled the teachers to continue blaming them for their lack of involvement. It also left teachers unable to examine how the school, and they themselves, contributed to the problems.

The focus on problem students or parental failure obscured the fact that the various problems in attendance, dropouts, violence and disrupted classes were symptoms rather than disease. They were reactions to membership in a large urban school in which individuals felt lost and disconnected, isolated and bored, and alienated (Zane 1994). Students were expressing themselves, if artlessly, making others feel scared, angry, and upset; hopeless and despairing; intruded upon; rejected. They were communicating as best they could through the wordless process of projective identification. Thurston teachers and administrators received those messages – they felt what their students felt – but were unable or unwilling to decipher their meanings. They simply coded them in terms of the students' being out of control.

These perceptions enabled teachers and administrators to avoid examining how Thurston itself was out of control. The school was, in point of fact, a series of disjointed programs: special education programs, multiple tracks, advanced classes. The school was fragmented, split into pieces that held little relation to one another. The staff were fragmented as well. Teachers were split off from the administrators, each blaming the other for the state of the school. Teachers were split off from one another, located as they were in different departments, programs, and tracks. Their splits fell along identity group lines, with the minority teachers connecting more with one another than with their white colleagues, and vice versa, much like the student cliques.

These splits were not publicly discussed at Thurston. Nor was the general sense that the school was out of control, spinning out different, disconnected programs with little guiding vision. It was incumbent upon the students, as the politically weakest group in the school, to express indirectly what could not be expressed directly. They acted out their alienated responses. They were, after a fashion, messengers bent on delivering news to the school about itself. They were also its casualties.

Community Groups

A small group of Thurston administrators and teachers working with a consultant created a program called "Community Groups." Education research suggested that small educational communities enhance teachers' professional development, parents' levels of involvement, and students' academic and social outcomes (Fine 1994). The program involved assigning teachers to cohorts of students. These Community Groups would meet weekly together. Their task involved simply talking about issues that students wished to address. Such issues ranged widely, from school policies and teacher-student relations to situations involving peer pressure, drugs, teenage pregnancy, and other trials of an urban adolescence. Community Groups were designed to form meaningful attachments between adolescents and adults, on the premise that such relationships enable students to express and work through obstacles to academic and social achievement. These relationships were meant to last: Community Groups were to meet for four years, enabling students and staff to create sustained relationships.

The Community Group program at Thurston also implicitly represented an intervention in the teachers' social defense system. Their defenses were sustained by remaining distant from the personal lives of their students, and Community Groups pressed them right up against those personal lives. Teachers' projections and stereotypes would be burst by knowing students as persons (Powell 1994). The Community Groups program legitimated conversations about racism, accountability, and the societal violence that flooded public schools (Fine 1994). Such conversations represented a bringing in rather than a pushing away of the urban environment so deeply embedded within the students. The students themselves were brought closer to the adults in the school. In such programs, Powell (1994: 120) notes, "Students feel known in a deeper way and are less likely to disappear because they feel unnoticed." They are able to safely express and explore difficult feelings and master them in adaptive ways.

The Community Groups program thus represented an intervention in teachers' relations with one another and with school administrators. Working in pairs with their assigned student cohorts, they needed to engage with one another rather then remain isolated. The program required them to plan, reflect, and build curriculum together. It required them to support one another during difficult conversations and build upon one another's ideas. It required them, ideally, to draw upon their personal selves in their work (Kahn 1992), which meant sharing feelings and reactions, personal experiences, and reflections on their own biases and projections. Teachers were implicitly being asked to disassemble their defenses against attaching both to the students and to one another.

The launch

Teachers had varying reactions to the Community Groups program. A number of senior teachers were uninterested. They believed that the program would inevitably follow the same path of similar others: announced to great fanfare and promises, implemented in a few high-profile classrooms, given little resources or administrative support, and finally allowed to fade away once it was unable to produce short-term results on standardized scores, parental satisfaction, and other measures that mattered to the school super-intendent and local administrators. These senior teachers were jaded and cynical. Some of them had allowed themselves to hope during previous interventions and had been sorely disappointed. They were determined not to allow themselves to be hurt in such ways again.

Other teachers newer to the school or simply more willing to risk disap-pointment liked the promise of the Community Groups program. They were encouraged that Thurston's vice-principal rather than the superintendent's office, which was viewed with some mistrust, had generated the program. These teachers perceived Community Groups as a way to do something small yet significant in the face of the crushing urban blight affecting their students. They were eager to relate more deeply with students. A third group of teachers, constituting the majority, were unsure about the program and their involve-ment. They occupied a large middle ground: aware that the school needed some significant change, hoping this program might be that change, but waiting to invest their own energies until it seemed clear that it would work. This group remained poised between the other two, watching and waiting.

Thurston's vice-principal brought together a committee of teachers to design the program. On the advice of the consultant the committee was explicitly diverse, along various dimensions: commitment to an intervention; seniority; race, ethnicity, and gender. The committee was to develop the process by which Community Groups was to be introduced to teachers, administrators, and students and implemented across the school. The committee met weekly throughout a school year in anticipation of introducing the program to teachers and administrators at the end of the year, providing training over the summer, and implementing the program at the beginning of the following year.

It became clear during those weekly meetings that the Community Groups program threatened to disturb a set of entrenched teacher interests. Some teachers were determined not to lose their autonomy. They believed that the Community Groups program would inevitably encroach on their abilities to decide what, when and how to raise issues with students. The vice-principal made it clear that this was indeed likely to be the case: teachers would have to collaborate in the design and conduct of the program, and students were likely to raise issues that would take both the Community Groups and regular classroom discussions in unpredictable directions. The vice-principal emphasized that it made little sense to offer students the opportunity to raise issues and then severely limit what, when, and how they were able to discuss them.

Another coalition of teachers on the committee made clear their wishes not to work with students who were not in the more advanced tracks. These teachers had always had seniority within the school, enabling them to teach only advance track students. The Community Groups program involved creating heterogeneous groups that cut across various tracks. Thurston had devolved into a caste society based on tracks, with relations between students from different tracks marked by projections and stereotypes. Many of the teachers themselves, particularly those that worked solely with the advance track students, propagated those projections and stereotypes, which drove their resistance to the Community Groups program. The vice-principal countered by suggesting that seniority might no longer guarantee the assignment of teachers to specific tracks and levels.

There were also the entrenched interests of teachers who differed in racial identity. As the planning of the Community Groups program grew more detailed and the conversations among the planning group became more revealing, it emerged that white teachers and teachers of color by and large approached the students differently. The white teachers had relatively low academic expectations for students of color, compared to the teachers of color. They graded students of color more leniently, on the premise that "they're doing the best they can do." They challenged those students less and in turn received less from those students, which seemed to confirm the white teachers' perceptions. This angered the teachers of color on the planning committee, who accused the white teachers of racism. They accused them of preparing students of color only for minimum-wage jobs and unfulfilling lives. The teachers of color also discovered differences among themselves: some believed that the bar should be lowered for students of color, who struggled daily with urban afflictions, while others argued that such an approach simply kept students trapped in cycles of poverty and despair.

The committee grew paralyzed by its accumulated differences. Members were silent, unsure of how to address the issues. Or they raged at one another, leveling accusations that did little to encourage empathy and awareness. The committee remained thus, veering between fight and flight, for several weeks. Finally, several of them were able to hear and work effectively with the consultant to understand the underlying dynamics at play. They were able to understand how their struggles paralleled those in the larger school, and moreover, in the larger community. The consultant and vice-principal emphasized to them that they were not expected to solve these issues. They were simply to design a process whereby the school's wider community of teachers, administrators, and ultimately students were able to learn about and implement the new program.

To remain stuck in the fight or flight patterns of discussion would, the consultant argued, maintain the status quo in the teachers' relations with one another and with their students. It would maintain the defenses that marked how they avoided meaningful relations, at cost to themselves and to their students. The committee ultimately accepted this. With some difficulty, members stayed with the task of designing the Community Groups program, figuring out logistics, training, and curricula. They launched the program the following fall, after conducting introductory training workshops for faculty and students.

Success and failure

The Community Groups program was greeted by the Thurston community of teachers and students with a mixture of interest, cynicism, and caution. The initial training workshops helped staff and students understand the purposes, design, and intended process of the Community Groups. A school assembly heralded the beginning, with supportive remarks by the principal and several students and teachers from another school that had implemented a similar program. The school broke into the new groupings, teachers and students warily entering new rooms and roles with one another.

The first month of Community Group meetings was marked by both uncertainty and valid attempts by both teachers and students. Each group engaged in a certain amount of testing: the students were testing to see how safe it was to speak openly without censure or ridicule while the teachers struggled to respond in ways that demonstrated their acceptance of the students and the process. All were searching for ways to be participants and facilitators while remaining aware of their ongoing roles outside the Community Groups.

The initial success or failure of particular Community Groups was largely related to individual teachers' abilities to manage boundaries: beginning and ending on time, enforcing stable membership, keeping conversations on track, managing conflict among students, encouraging respectful discourse. When the teachers were able to manage such boundaries their students felt safe enough to become increasingly open and authentic. This was particularly true when these teachers themselves responded thoughtfully to student concerns without becoming disabled by affect, their own or that of the students. They managed to take in and digest students' anxiety without becoming undone by it; they created holding environments (Kahn 2001). The less successful Community Groups were characterized by various disruptions of holding environments. Students wandered in and out, treated one another and the teachers disrespectfully, were superficial and dismissive, or simply withdrew. These teachers were unable to fully assume an effective facilitator role.

The Community Groups were haunted by racial politics similar to those that beset the planning committee. Students of color raged against the white society that "kept them down" while at the same time labeling themselves as powerless victims, "and nothing we can do about it." White students, for their part, expressed little anger but spoke of the unfairness of teachers who did not seem to let them off easy and of how hard they had to work for what they had. In the initial stages of the Community Groups, cross-race conversations about drugs, violence, sex, and achievement were often in the language of stereotypes. White students implied that students of color were angry, violent, academic failures. Students of color implied that white students were privileged, colorless, protected. These implications hovered over the groups, impeding students' conversations and connections.

The teachers received additional training to deal with racial issues. They were asked to examine their own racial identities and beliefs, which some did with greater reflection and insight than others. Some understood that a sea of projections and stereotypes that existed within the larger society and were imported into the school by students, teachers, and administrators created the racial gulfs at Thurston. A few were able to take that understanding back into their groups and help students become more aware of when and why they were using stereotypes. Other teachers were unable to offer such insights; their groups remained more or less paralyzed by ongoing conflict or by student withdrawal and boredom.

It was a more difficult proposition to deal with the parents of some of the advanced-track students. They resisted the idea of heterogeneous community groups and complained to the principal. They argued that their children had little to learn from other students who had little academic interest or aptitude, were into drugs or gangs, or who disengaged from the activities and attitudes of the "normal, high achiever" students. The principal listened closely to them. While he supported, in theory, the Community Groups program, he also felt pressure to maintain separate elite tracks to attract "good" students.

Academically high-achieving students produced high standardized test scores, which constituted one of the measures by which the school and its administrators were evaluated. The principal did not wish to alienate the parents of students producing high scores. Nor did he wish to alienate the administrators, teachers, and students who were beginning to value the Community Groups program.

The principal remained torn between these competing interests until the district superintendent forced his hand near the end of the first year of the program. Several parents of Thurston students had complained to the superintendent's office about what they were hearing from their children about Community Groups. The parents were offended by student discussions of teenage sex, peer pressure, and drugs. The superintendent passed the complaints along to the principal, advising him to halt the program or curtail it sharply. The principal held a series of meetings with his staff and the teachers over the summer to discuss the program. The vice-principal argued that they needed to see the program's effects on outcome measures before any decisions about its future were made. The principal said that, as far as he and the superintendent were concerned, the results were in. With much dissension and difficulty the principal decided to discontinue the program. The vice-principal soon after tendered his resignation and took a job in another school district.

Care versus control

Had the Community Groups program at Thurston continued and its outcomes been evaluated, there would very likely have been the types of positive result found in similar programs. Such programs can effectively interrupt the social defenses that keep teachers and students from meaningful relationships (Fine 1994; Powell 1994). They begin to know one another, moving past superficial categories and labels and into meaningful attachments. This has resulted in reduced violence in some schools, gradual de-emphasis of disciplinary issues, and valuing of academic learning and achievement. As Zane (1994: 123) notes, the "fetish with disciplinary concerns diminishes as schools ... become more relationally oriented." Teachers advocate for, rather than simply discipline, students. They heighten their expectations of all students and all students strive to satisfy rather than disappoint those expectations. They develop educational partnerships with students, distributing the responsibility for student learning. Students act out less, become less violent, show up for class, and do their work (Fine 1994).

To have sustained the Community Groups program at Thurston and achieved such outcomes, the principal would have had to have the political will to see each and every child develop to the peak of his or her capacities (Fine 1994). He would have had to be able to withstand assaults from teachers who did not wish to teach lower-level tracks, parents whose children were in advanced tracks, and a district superintendent who wanted no political disturbances. He would also have had to struggle against the incentive systems that tied his rewards to student achievement measured by standardized tests. The concern was not simply that parents of high-achieving students would remove them from the school. More insidious, it was that if the Community Groups program was effective, the dropout rate would lower, and with it the average test scores for the school. The incentive system was thus implicitly tied to weaker students having fewer attachments to the school and leaving.

The politics surrounding the struggle over the implementation and survival of the Community Groups were both internal and external. Teachers with entrenched interests in working with advance-track students were aligned with the parents of those students; neither wanted close contact with students considered troubled or undesirable. They in turn represented a larger piece of society that wished to maintain the separation between "normal, high-achieving" people and the "others," those steeped in crime, drugs, poverty, and other urban ills (a separation that society often manages through the incarceration of those "others"). Similarly, the white teachers and teachers of color struggling over expectations of students of color represented a societal struggle over responsibility and accountability. Society itself is torn between the image of students of color as victims or as personally responsible. The struggles of everyone – students, teachers, parents, school administrators – with Community Groups, standardized tests, and the tracks were waged on behalf of a larger society wishing to resolve larger questions of responsibility and hopelessness.

The school's politics also represented another battle endemic to caregiving organizations: to *care for* versus *control* careseekers. To *care* for others is to tend to them personally and individually; to bring them in and digest their needs; to hold them as they need to be held. To *control* others is to ensure that they follow prescribed systems and procedures through which the organization delivers its services. While the two are not by definition incompatible, in practice they often exist as such. Caring for Thurston students would involve a school pointed toward fully developing the capacities of *all* students. Controlling them meant creating multiple tracks, labeling and categorizing students into those tracks, and developing curricula that fitted those categories. Caring occurs in the context of meaningful relationships and attachments. Control occurs in the context of systems and processes that maintain distance between people in different roles. The district superintendent, who insisted upon maintaining the status quo, and the principal who went along with him, emphasized control over care.

Of course, controlling careseekers is also in the service of their care. Control enables the long-term viability of caregiving organizations. Without structures and systems that regulate the flow of patients into and through hospital departments, the filling of beds in residential care, and the scheduling of school classes and activities, these organizations would be filled with chaos. Anarchy would ensue. Boundaries would be too permeable. Careseekers and caregivers would flail about, unsure of where they ought to be and what they ought to be doing. On the other hand, control can be overemphasized, and too often is. Standardized testing forces teacher-student interactions to conform to certain specifications that produce specific outcomes. The unvarying routines of many nursing homes, residential treatment centers, and long-term care facilities manage populations rather than care for individual patients. The vast amount of paperwork that social workers and healthcare workers complete that requires them to label and fit clients into pre-existing categories masks the individual ways in which each client cannot be so categorized.

When the control of careseekers takes precedence over their care, much as when the disciplining of students takes precedence over their learning, social defenses are often at play. At Thurston High School the emphasis on controlling students was intimately related to their anonymity. Teachers knew students not as individuals but as an unruly mass, prone to violence that needed to be suppressed before it exploded. The students by and large remained faceless. This enabled teachers and administrators to defend against the anxiety, sadness, guilt, anger, and other emotions triggered by the urban poverty their students so acutely represented. The social defense system created casualties. Students remained anonymous, unattached to responsive, caring teachers. Teachers who wished for such relationships were disappointed as well. They withdrew from students and one another, grew cynical and hopeless. Administrators were forced to preside over battles and war zones rather than create climates for teaching and learning. The school itself was a casualty.

The failure of Thurston to create an ultimately successful intervention, in the form of Community Groups, was also related to widespread if covert beliefs about the school and its students. The district superintendent, principal, and complaining parents of advance-track students were likely influenced by societal projections about most urban school students as inferior, violent, dangerous, and hopeless. In the light of those beliefs the decision to halt a program designed to help "normal" students voice troubling issues and thereby create both the space and relationships for learning to occur is understandable, if reprehensible. These students were not considered "normal." They were assumed to be inferior. This assumption enabled other parts of society to consider themselves superior, and competent, relative to urban schools, which fall into what Powell and Barber (2004) term the "politics of despair." The politics surrounding the introduction, launch, and dismantling of the Thurston Community Groups program were marked by such despair. They occurred within a swirl of unspoken projections about the students and the groups they represented within the larger society.

Inside out

Caregiving organizations routinely represent societal issues. Like vessels they contain the mix of issues, fears, hopes, and anxieties triggered by the tasks they perform on behalf of the societies in which they are embedded. They become microcosms of society, their varying (and vying) groups recreated within the organizations themselves. There is often enough little distinction between caregiving organizations and their environments, as people flow across relatively permeable boundaries. It is in this context that caregiving organizations and their members must accomplish their tasks of teaching, healing, growing, or caring for others.

Altering the contexts themselves – society and its institutions – is not a viable strategy. The teachers at Thurston are not likely to alter the flow of white students into the suburbs, the homelessness and poverty of their students of color, the constant images on television and other media that fuel societal splitting and projections along the lines of race and class, or the insistence on standardized testing as the measure of all students' abilities and futures. This is not to suggest that those teachers or caregiving organization members more generally are helpless. On the contrary: they have a great opportunity to alter what occurs within their boundaries.

To do so, they must quite explicitly understand that their organizations are microcosms of the societies in which they are embedded. Members must be consciously aware that larger forces influence them. They must deliberately seek to interpret and interrupt the destructive impact of those larger forces, by working with what they have been given: a society in miniature over which they have some control. If they are able to resolve the issues in that miniature society, they can affect the larger environment, in the way that a pebble dropped into a still pond can send small ripples to its edges. With enough pebbles, ripples become waves. An example can be found in Powell's (1997) account of creating a classroom in which teachers and students examined the academic performance and experience of white students and students of color. The students' experiences of such a classroom are carried with them into, and shape their actions within, their school more generally. Societies change in such ways, from the inside out.

At Thurston, teachers and administrators had before them a re-creation of the society in which they lived and worked. They regarded that miniature society with a mixture of fear, anger, frustration, and denial. They saw only the dilemma of how to educate an urban population. There is another framing: the opportunity to work with the issues that students present – homelessness, family or community violence, learning difficulties, cultural differences – in the service of the education task (Fine 1994). In practice, this means framing educational tasks partly in terms of applying academic concepts to the material represented by the real lives of students. At Thurston, for example, teachers would develop a curriculum based on applying various disciplines to the urban environment of their students. Economics, mathematics, history, social studies, literature: all could find expression and meaning in the context of studying the urban blight that gave rise to the distress that the students daily carried with them into their school. The students would have reasons to consider academic material relevant to their lives, rather than as simply another trial not of their choosing that they must endure.

Engaging this task requires people to work together amidst a great deal of anxiety that will get stirred up by looking at rather than ignoring distressing circumstances. Teachers will need to work together in departments or project teams to create curricula. Principals will need to fight the political battles that will inevitably emerge, as resources are invested in bringing the real lives of students and academic material in closer relation to one another, and not incidentally, as a school attempts to cater to all students rather than simply those slotted into advanced tracks. Teachers and students will, finally, need to allow themselves to move closer toward one another if each is to learn from and teach one another as their worlds collide. They will need to zealously protect the boundaries around what occurs in their classrooms if they are to have a chance of leaning in toward one another.

Chapter 10

Running in place

Organizational life involves periods of progress and change and periods of idling within the status quo. Progress is marked by decisions made and acted upon. Strategies are developed and implemented. Leaders are authorized and followed. Relations within and between groups improve, releasing energy within individuals and organizations that gets channeled into their tasks. People discuss, confront, engage, and address issues preventing them from working together effectively. New ground is explored. This contrasts with periods of "stuckness." People create repetitive, ineffective patterns. Decisions are not made or made but not acted upon. Committees meet, make recommendations, and disband without changing anything. Departments maintain uneasy alliances or awkward distances. Systems and processes remain in place even though they are clearly ineffectual or damaging. People leave themselves mired in these patterns.

Stuckness is inevitable in social systems. Indeed, the development of relationships, groups, and organizations is characterized by cycles of movement and stuckness (Smith & Berg 1987). People routinely find themselves stuck, caught in patterns that frustrate them and their capacities to do what they wish to do. Social systems develop when people take risks – trusting others, making themselves vulnerable, raising difficult issues – that enable them to figure out what lies beneath frustrating patterns and act accordingly. This occurs over and again, as people move ahead and then press up against further limits in their relationships. These limits manifest differently in different social systems. In a marriage one partner might keep pushing unsuccessfully for more intimacy. A group might find itself unable to authorize any of its members to lead. An organization may be marked by constant battles between two divisions whose leaders cannot reconcile their differences. People may remain caught in such ineffective patterns, or they may explore issues underlying those patterns (Smith & Berg 1987). If they choose the latter their relationships, groups and organizations keep developing. They get stuck and then they move, leading to further stuckness and further movement, *ad infinitum*.

In some organizations, as in some relationships and groups, movement does not occur. People remain caught in ineffective patterns of working and relating. They are left running in place, with lots of activity and pressure but little forward movement. There are various ways to understand this. The history of an organization may prevent its members from changing. A founder's death might leave organization members unable or unwilling to disturb the status quo. Outdated strategies may hold sway, and potential leaders who could move the organization towards more effective strategies are discouraged from doing so. An organization's culture may prevent its members from openly confronting ineffective structures, policies, or intergroup relations. Another's culture may emphasize blame and risk avoidance. Overly bureaucratic or punitive systems may prevent organization members from providing leaders with candid assessments. Members may work in an industry or organization that eschews reflecting on their work processes. Any of these or similar factors may help to explain organizations that remain unalterably stuck.

Caregiving organizations are unique to the extent that their stuckness is so often set or kept in motion by *trauma* of one sort or another. Such trauma may be direct and acute, an episode that erupts within one part of the organization and like an earthquake strikes a target and disrupts the surrounding areas. It may be direct and chronic, as caregivers experience trauma in relations with careseekers. It may be vicarious, created by constant exposure to careseekers' traumas. In any of these forms, trauma seeps into caregiving organizations and affects not only those involved but the organizations as well. It becomes an underlying dis-ease whose primary symptom is ongoing organizational stuckness.

Organizational trauma

The most obvious source of trauma in caregiving organizations is violent episodes that occur within their boundaries. A student stabs another at school. Gang members fight in a neighborhood social service agency. A social worker commits suicide in her office. A hospital patient dies from a medication error. A patient assaults a clerical worker at a health clinic. A minister is publicly accused of sexual abuse. A violent patient sexually threatens a nurse. Such episodes erupt within caregiving organizations and assault those who are at their epicenter and, inevitably, radiate out to other organization members.

Trauma in caregiving organizations may also be cumulative and relatively subtler. Students routinely verbally assault teachers in an urban school. Childcare workers at a residential treatment center are kicked and spat upon during physical restraints. Frustrated, frightened patients and their families verbally harass nurses in an emergency room. Residents working the psychiatric ward of a teaching hospital are daily confronted by unruly patients seeking immediate release or help. While none of these patterns may erupt in a traumatic event *per se*, their cumulative effects can over time induce within caregivers and other organization members a sense of being traumatized. They may become shell-shocked by the constant assault. They may, like trauma victims, feel helpless and terrified, over time rather than all of a sudden.

Trauma in caregiving organizations may be vicarious as well. Secondary traumatic stress affects caregivers who work with others and "soak up" their emotional pain (Figley 1995). Like soldiers who witness much violence and death, and develop battle fatigue, caregivers exposed to much abuse and pain develop compassion fatigue. Social workers and childcare workers who work with child abuse victims may be traumatized by their intimate exposure to that abuse. Nurses, physicians, and support staff working a burn unit, pediatric cancer ward or AIDS facility may feel the trauma of their patients and their families. Crisis workers, disaster relief workers, and emergency medical technicians who work the sites of natural disasters, terrorism and large-scale accidents may be secondarily traumatized by close contact with the victims' trauma. The toxicity of such secondary traumatic stress for caregivers may equal that of post-traumatic stress for the trauma victims themselves.

Trauma affects individuals in powerful ways. Past trauma may profoundly affect how people experience current situations. Trauma victims relive the event, wishing to master the feelings it aroused, largely to no avail; they continue to feel terror, rage, and helplessness. They experience difficulty in maintaining close relationships. These symptoms often remain even while trauma events seemingly fade; indeed, they may become disconnected from their originating sources (Herman 1997). When individuals are able to develop effective therapeutic relationships they are able to process their trauma, reconnect their symptoms to their sources, and eventually dismiss their symptoms as no longer vital for their healthy functioning.

Trauma affects organizations as well as individuals. Caregiving organizations whose members have pronounced, ongoing difficulty in maintaining useful working relationships may be understood as traumatized. Trauma can be collective; it can be a property of the organization itself, or of specific units, not simply of individual members. When violent or traumatic episodes erupt in caregiving organizations they dramatically affect those closest in proximity, just as traumatized careseekers affect caregivers who work most closely with them. Trauma then radiates throughout caregiving organizations. Caregivers interact with one another, administrators and staff, they communicate not simply information but emotional experiences. Other organization members thus experience vicariously that which was first borne by whoever was at the epicenter of traumatic episodes or accumulations. There is a ripple effect resulting in waves of secondary traumatization. Organizations can thus be wounded, and their members' sense of safety and identity disrupted, regardless of whether any particular individual suffered personal losses (Myers & Wee 2002).

Caregiving organizations thus become repositories for trauma. If they are able to process the trauma, organizations and their members can integrate painful experiences into daily functioning without being unduly disabled (Dutton 2003; Frost 2003). If they are unable to process the trauma it seeps into the organization itself. There it remains, disturbing the organization's functioning like bodily waste that cannot be flushed out of the human system. The organization develops symptoms disconnected from the trauma itself and these may function as social defenses, unconsciously developed to distract members from the trauma and its suppressed pain. Like individual defenses against trauma, these social defenses assume lives of their own. And like individual defenses, the social defenses inevitably call attention to rather than suppress trauma.

In this chapter I illustrate how an organization becomes stuck in ineffective patterns grounded in unresolved trauma. The illustration comes from an action research project I completed with hospital operating room staff seeking to improve work and working relations. This chapter contains information originally reported in Kahn (2003).

Maple Hospital surgical unit

Maple Hospital was located in Maple Heights, a middle-class, blue-collar city of 100,000. Its community hospital had over the years lost a great many patients to the sprawling university hospital located 30 miles away, which held the promise of the latest academic research and medical procedures. The elderly patients remained loyal. Maple Hospital was where they and their children were born, where their parents were cared for and where some of them worked. It was their children, the more entitled and demanding consumers, who were leading the exodus to the university hospital or to hospitals in nearby affluent communities that boasted newer facilities. To compete, Maple had to create a number of specialized services and a reputation for outstanding care. It had to bring in physicians and their patients, who would bring insurers and money.

The hospital was perched high on a hill overlooking the city. Its physical plant was serviceable, in the way of an old high school, with worn linoleum floors, cranky elevators, and stucco walls. Built in the early 1900s, it was at one time the city's jewel. That time had long passed. "The city raped the place for years," a surgeon who had practiced there for 30 years said. "The money went to the city. The contracts to run and fix the place went to the mayor's cronies. For years the wind rattled through the windows." In the surgical unit (SU) space was tight, not so much in the operating rooms but in the pre- and postoperative areas where patients had little privacy, often separated by nothing more than a drawn curtain that did nothing to stop them from hearing the details of one another's procedures and conversations. Money was tight too, for purchasing new equipment that would entice surgeons practicing elsewhere and for hiring more staff.

The SU had recently acquired a new chief of surgery, Dr Palmer. He was hired to help turn the unit around. He had discovered in his first three months that his influence over some of the forces shaping patient volume – referrals from primary care physicians, influxes of new surgeons and their business – depended on his ability to create a unit to which people wanted to come. The unit he had inherited was not that. It was too ill for that, with a disease that presented itself in how people worked together. "The unit has zero team-work," Dr Palmer said. "It's pretty much everyone for themselves. Everybody has his own agenda, often in conflict with one another. It's not about pulling together." He wanted to change how unit members worked together:

> This place is like the Wild, Wild West. They make up the rules as they go along and then change them to suit their fancy. They don't trust one another. It's a dysfunctional family. I've got surgeons venting in front of patients, berating staff, who retaliate by slowing down and being unaccommodating. I've got staff nurses who won't go out of their way to help new surgeons who represent new business. People here are just not collegial. Their first instinct is to blame.

I conducted an organizational diagnosis of the SU over the course of six months, with observations and interviews culminating in a series of feed-back meetings with organization members. The themes presented below were part of the feedback material.

On the edge

The SU was at a particularly difficult point in its history. Patient volume was low. The unit was understaffed. Personnel had left and not been replaced, leaving the remaining nurses and technicians overworked and the operating rooms underutilized. It was difficult to increase patient volume given the focus on cost-cutting measures that reduced customers for all hospitals. Patients had more choices and were attracted to competitors with good facilities and management. The Maple Hospital administration had not been proactive in developing and promoting a public marketing strategy to attract patients. Primary care physicians were referring patients to other hospitals, or keeping them out of hospitals altogether, because they lacked confidence in the Maple Hospital SU or because of financial incentives from insurance companies. Surgeons were also opting to practice elsewhere. They found more service-oriented SU leadership and staff, more accommodating scheduling, better equipment, more fully stocked supplies, and less restrictive rules and procedures in other hospitals. The Maple Hospital SU was struggling for its survival.

Rather than pulling together to work with their leaders to create a unit to which surgeons and patients wanted to come, SU members pulled apart from one another. Distracting sub-groups marked the unit. There were groups of nurses and surgeons who supported or opposed the nurse manager; nurses who supported or opposed the union; surgeons who supported or opposed Dr Palmer's emphasis on customer satisfaction. The SU also functioned on the basis of overly personal relationships. People made decisions (e.g., nurse managers' scheduling of cases and shifts, surgeons' requests for specific nurses) and reacted to one another (e.g., feedback or requests for assistance) on the basis of the history of their personal relationships with one another. SU personnel focused on their personal agendas. They sought control of their incomes, schedules, territories, and job descriptions, and protected themselves from others, undermining their abilities to work together effectively.

Various members and leaders of the unit had in previous years suggested various ways to improve the unit's functioning, to little avail. They had requested additional resources, most particularly personnel who would ease the burden on existing staff and enable the opening of more operating rooms. They had tried to create new systems for coordinating patient flow, replenishing supplies and equipment, and holding people accountable for effective job performance. They had tried to replace individuals in nursing leadership, staff or physician roles who could not work effectively with others. These attempts had failed, partly because the SU lacked the capacity to solve problems together. Leaders and members had not been able to pursue a common vision for creating a viable, thriving unit.

Nurse manager, lightning rod

The nurse manager, Barbara Nash, emerged as a lightning rod attracting the heat and light of the unit's energy. Barbara had worked at the hospital for almost 30 years, the last twelve as SU nurse manager. She ran the unit's daily operations: she scheduled surgeries, assigned shifts, hired and trained nurses and technicians, maintained the unit budget, and worked with the chief of surgery to ensure smooth relations between her staff and the surgeons. She had a great deal of power, over her staff, whom she hired, fired, scheduled, and managed, and over the surgeons, scheduling their regular operating times and their "add-ons," emergent cases that required surgery within a day.

In the interviews, people kept circling back to Barbara as if she occupied a central zone they must constantly traverse. Many perceived her as playing favorites with nurses and surgeons. She rewarded nurses she liked, they said, with desirable shifts and hours while treating others disrespectfully. "She treats some nurses like children," said one, "even calling them dodo. And she yells at them in front of others." Surgeons reported that Barbara rewarded those she liked with desirable schedules, quick add-ons, and good nurses.

"She makes some surgeons' lives miserable," one said. "Its selective suffering," said another. "She knows how to work the system, and no one has the balls to get her out. She's called a senior surgeon an asshole to his face and Dr Palmer one behind his back." They tell many stories about her rudeness. Barbara also had her defenders, who saw her as a victim of sorts, blamed by surgeons who disliked the paperwork or safety procedures that she enforced or by pro-union nurses for whom she represented hospital administration.

Barbara framed her leadership differently. "I'm not going to please people," she said. "It's part of the job." The divisions in the unit, she said, were there because of the unions. "It's hard to motivate the staff because they're entitled, saying 'it's not my job.' Some of us fight that and others resent it." Barbara believed that some of the surgeons resented her because she was a stickler for the procedures that ensured safety. "I make sure that patients go safely through the system. The physicians just want to get the job done, and don't spend enough time with the patients." She believed that she was forced into various battles, with nurses swayed by the union or with surgeons who placed their own convenience above the safety of their patients. She saw herself as the guardian of the hospital and its patients. She wished for a less embattled unit but was unaware of how her own style – favoring allies and punishing enemies – helped draw the very battle lines demarcating the unit.

Barbara was clearly a divisive force in the unit, whose members rallied for or against but not around her as a respected leader. She was unable to instill teamwork and collegiality in the unit. The question was why she was retained as nurse manager. There were a number of immediate possible answers. She kept costs low and worked within tight budgets. Her boss, the recently fired vice-president of nursing, had protected her because she defended patients (against the surgeons) and the administration (against the unionized nurses). The hospital administrators were also busy with difficult financial and strategic issues.

None of these explanations, however, addressed why the hospital administration *wanted* an SU marked by conflict and dissension. Like most organizations, Maple Hospital had a thriving grapevine; the various senior administrators during the last decade had certainly heard the stories about Barbara's leadership. They must also have known that there were other nurse managers able to work within tight budgets and encourage teamwork, even in unionized environments. They must also have known that the potential costs of conflict among SU staff would be catastrophic: a misinterpreted word here or a shrug of the shoulder there and the wrong dosage or drug or X-ray would go unchecked, with real consequences for patients. In spite of such potential consequences, Barbara remained the nurse manager. This kept the unit's conflicts in place in spite of the damage to the SU. It was as if Barbara was a key part of some sort of defense mechanism for the hospital or the SU. The question was, what were they defending against?

The event

During the organizational diagnosis, surgeons and nurses referred to a particular surgical error in the Maple SU. Some referred to it in passing, obliquely, while for others it occupied a more central place. Five years earlier, a surgeon had badly botched an operation, removing the wrong internal organ. There were various versions of the story. One blamed the surgeon. "The appropriate diagnostic information was on the chart and there was verification in the room," Barbara Nash said. "But the surgeon just took over and made an assumption." Another version blamed Barbara herself for not requiring the surgeon to follow standard operating procedures, such as having X-rays and charts in the room, because he was one of her favorites. The surgeon himself reported, "It was a screw up of a whole bunch of things." He listed them: "The patient was already in the room but none of the films were. I didn't know I could access them there. I had the patient confused in my mind with another patient. It had been seven or eight weeks since I had seen the patient. I didn't have access to my own notes. And I was rushed to get out of the room by other doctors." He portrayed himself as out of the loop, hurriedly operating in the dark.

The patient survived, the lawsuit was quietly settled, and the surgeon and his assistant, after being suspended and put on probation, still practiced at Maple. There were state and national investigations. Maple Hospital was required to develop and implement an action plan based on a thorough analysis of what had gone wrong. The event was picked up first by the local newspaper, which ran a number of articles on the error, and then nationally. Suddenly Maple Hospital was notorious. It became a lightning rod for people's terror about being defenseless on an operating table and having someone make an awful mistake that was at once ludicrous and preventable. The press fed the terror. A surgeon noted, "The newspapers made it sound moronic, as if the surgeons were just stupid. The operation had some degree of difficulty. Yes, it was clearly a bad mistake. But the press portrayed them as bloodthirsty savages." "They were treated like criminals," said another surgeon of his colleagues. "They were at the wrong place at the wrong time."

The Maple SU surgeons and staff felt that way about themselves as well. "Look," a senior physician said, "this kind of thing, or errors of equally bad culpability, happens all the time at lots of hospitals. It's just not reported at most places." Medical errors are traditionally handled internally with reviews, action plans, and where appropriate, sanctions. "Who called the paper?" the assisting surgeon said, still aggrieved at the betrayal five years later. "We felt like they were bullying the weak local community hospital," reported a nurse. The unit as a whole felt victimized. The publicity left the SU staff reeling.

They were also left with no place to turn. Unit members were told by hospital administrators not to talk about the event. There was no public discussion. "We discussed it at grand rounds a month later," recalled one surgeon. "Meanwhile," she continued, "a murmur went around and around until it became a scream." The scream was ignored. "No one," a nurse said, "came and talked with us, said this is okay, it happens other places, we'll get through it. We were told to keep quiet. We were even threatened by the management." Another said, "No one ever came up and said, you've had a tough time, asked how we're doing. It was all about confidentiality, don't say a word to anyone about anything. Don't talk in the elevator and at lunch where people can hear you." The embattled administrators, trying to control the media coverage, public perceptions, and potential lawsuits, demanded silence from the staff. SU members did not even speak openly with one another. They were left alone, by hospital administration and by one another.

The haunting

While there was no sustained, public discussion of the event and what it meant in the life of the SU, it remained alive within the unit. Its emotional traces lived within different individuals. Barbara cried during several conversations about the event. Several surgeons said they were still furious five years after the fact, with their colleagues or Barbara or the administration. A nurse and a surgeon reported recurring nightmares about mistakes and danger; one continued to be treated for depression triggered by the event. These were individual cases, yet they pointed to how emotions from the event – sadness, guilt, rage, and depression – remained alive in the unit, located within specific individuals.

The event also remained alive within the SU culture. Surgeons were now required to personally conduct patient histories and physicals on the day of surgery rather than rely on previous reports. The consent process involved multiple permission slips, insurance forms, and non-medical office visits between surgeons and their patients. Nurses checked surgeons' pre-op plans, verifying correct procedures and ensuring that they knew which operation was to be performed. This altered greatly the traditional power relationship between surgeons and nurses. Nurses reviewed surgeons' procedures and plans and were obliged to halt operations if specified procedures had not been followed.

Nurses were thus set up to protect the patients from the surgeons. The surgeons resented the implication. Their resentment surfaced in their chafing over pre-surgical procedures. "Barbara's fucking rules make it hard to get our cases done," one said. A less outraged surgeon noted, "Doctors don't like redundancy and don't think that the physicals are necessarily outdated after a week or a month. They resist, tossing charts back to the nurses or shouting at them." Nurses had little sympathy for the surgeons. "They created this mess," one said. "If we have to close the operating room because we're too strict and doing things right, so be it." They too resented the situation, for they had to not only police reluctant surgeons but deal with anxious patients, who said things to them like, "Don't take off the wrong leg, okay?" Both the nurses and the surgeons were stuck with identities they did not like.

They were also stuck with their resentment and anger. SU members had no place to discharge these emotions. Barbara Nash exacerbated rather than helped relieve these feelings by contributing to an atmosphere of blame and divisiveness. Indeed, she was a key part of the unit's social defenses, which depended on unit members remaining constantly upset and angry. This enabled members to avoid feeling sadness, guilt, loss, and vulnerability, which would have inevitably been part of their normal experiences of the event. As long as they were mad at one another they did not have to do the more difficult work of addressing the pain from the organizational trauma they experienced. Barbara Nash helped fracture the unit so members were constantly upset.

The SU was thus marked by a social defense preventing the excavation and cleansing of its wound. Barbara and her favoritism were simply a component of that mechanism. So was the ongoing blame and resentment that had sprung up around the safety procedures. So too was the unit's culture of self-protection. Each of these prevented SU members from working as a team, from being "collegial." Each was a defense against the possibility that they would get close enough to share their experiences of the event. The unit organized itself around a defense against the expression of emotions that had been suppressed for five years.

But the incident also remained alive in the unit. Like a finger pressing insistently on a wound, Barbara Nash maintained the pain from the incident. She tried to locate the pain in the surgeons, with whom she constantly battled. Her focus on compliance with safety rules was right and the surgeons knew that. But her belittling of them, publicly and to her nurses, was a constant reminder of the event for the whole unit. It was a punishment of the surgeons, which enabled unit members to believe that justice was being served. This too was part of the social defense system. As long as staff members accepted that the surgeons had been at fault and were being punished, they would not have to talk about their own experiences and feelings during and after the event.

Members thus acted out rather than spoke of their emotions. These emotions were kept alive for five years because they could not be fully buried, like disturbed ghosts that could not rest until what unsettled them was addressed, after which they could fade into the past where they belonged. The SU was haunted. Its members realized this, on some level of awareness, for they were asking for help. They wished for an exorcism. The unit's conflicts, blaming, lack of collegiality, and teamwork – all were smoke signals the unit unconsciously sent heavenward, looking for long-lost rescue.

Endgame

The SU feedback report focused on how the unit's informal sub-groups, overly personal relationships, and inability to work through the emotional, interpersonal and organizational implications of the incident five years earlier had prevented it from solving its own problems. The SU management team, which included Barbara Nash as well as Dr Palmer and the head of anesthesia, previewed the report before its distribution to the rest of the unit. The management team's conversation focused on the role that Barbara had played in the unit's dynamics. She seemed unaware of herself as a divisive figure in the unit. "It is not clear to people here," Dr Palmer told her, "whether you are able or willing to change who you are as a leader." She looked up. "Can I change?" she asked, as though thinking aloud. Dr Palmer answered, "I don't know whether or how you can change as quickly as we need you to." She looked at him, wanting a different response.

Several weeks later, Dr Palmer summoned Barbara to his office and offered her the choice to resign or be fired. She resigned, taking four months of paid leave. Dr Palmer was pleased, having discovered that there was little in her personnel file, in terms of performance reviews and disciplinary actions, to provide a paper trail justifying her dismissal. Previous senior administrators had ignored complaints about her: after putting out the gag order on the unit they had left it in place by the simple act of keeping Barbara just as she was. In leaving her there they had silenced the unit to protect the rest of the hospital.

Dr Palmer and other staff members believed that Barbara's departure solved the unit's problems. An interim nurse manager was hired. The staff liked her. She created transparently fair systems for surgeons and nurses and Dr Palmer reported that morale was high, noting, "The unit doesn't have people blaming one another as they once did." He and the interim nurse manager replaced 50 percent of the nurses and technicians. He also met regularly with the nurses every month or so to share information and listen to concerns. Over the year the SU had a few episodes of potential medical errors being caught at the last moment, one serious and the others less so. Dr Palmer reported they were handled well: reported, investigated, learned from, and dealt with. If true, this represented a move away from the old culture of blame.

On the face of it, the surgical model of identifying and removing "diseased" people seemingly solved the unit's issues. This goes directly against the therapeutic model underlying the notion of organizational trauma, which holds that unless underlying trauma is worked through, people and organizations cannot be fully resolved and functional. It is possible, of course, that removing both the scapegoat and half the staff interrupted the social defenses, as the people carrying the memory of the trauma were extruded. They became casualties, taking with them their pain like untreated trauma victims, and possibly leaving the remaining staff able to create new ways of relating.

It is also possible that the extrusions changed the surface but not the depth of the unit's work relationships. Indeed, once the interim nurse manager was replaced with the new permanent nurse manager, problems began to develop between her and a vocal cadre of nurses and surgeons involving issues of staff assignments. The unit also began to coalesce around its anger toward a senior technician who was perceived as sloppy in her work setting up for surgeries. The technician was not confronted, nor was her performance reviewed systematically. Each of these cases suggests the unit's ongoing capacity to focus on specific individuals as the cause of upset (i.e., to scapegoat) rather than on the larger underlying issues in the unit as a whole.

It may have also been too soon to tell whether or not the unit had indeed resolved its underlying issues. The extrusion of Barbara and other staff members did little to alter the unit's underlying capacities for managing traumatic experiences. The unit was not yet on safe ground. SU members and hospital leaders had not demonstrated the capacity to deal with the store of feelings that a serious medical error would release. They had not learned to talk in the midst of trauma, as they struggled with feelings of blame, rage, sadness, and guilt. They had not learned to refuse the gag order that inevitably gets issued at such times.

Principles of movement

Good therapists trace patterns of emotion to their sources. They look for underlying springs, some hole or wound in the individual from which the emotion originates. It is, often enough, some earlier trauma that went untreated. Children are emotionally and physically abused; siblings, parents, and lovers die; catastrophic accidents happen. Such traumas spawn sadness, rage, shame, guilt, and hurt. These emotions require direct expression. They need to be honored, talked about as if they matter, until people understand what they mean. If there is no place for this, people bury their emotions. They disconnect them from the traumas, which get forgotten or remembered in ways that may seem curiously dispassionate.

But trauma-induced emotions cannot be buried deeply enough. Like toxic waste they seep out. People unconsciously bootleg them into their current experiences. They unconsciously seek out and create situations that enable them to express buried emotions and they continue to do so until the original traumas are excavated and worked with in their proper context. Until that happens, the emotions take up a great deal of space in people's internal lives. The emotions and the events that spawned them are outsized, not yet placed in proper perspective.

Organizational units operate similarly. A combat unit gets ambushed and loses half its members. A small business goes bankrupt. An employee brings a gun and kills several colleagues before taking his own life. A beloved leader dies. A surgeon operates on the wrong organ and the local newspaper finds out. A priest sexually abuses boys and the Church hierarchy engages in a cover-up. These traumas affect the group, hitting some individuals harder or differently than others. The groups then contain the array of emotions triggered by the event: shock and disbelief; guilt about not preventing the event, and shame that it occurred at all; sadness and depression about loss; rage, at whatever or whoever seemed to cause the event. If people have places to talk about these emotions in the aftermath of the trauma they shared, the emotions are expressed and, over time, fade. If not, they lie pooled beneath the surface of people's interactions and seep out everywhere.

It is in exactly this way that organizations often break down and become stuck. Organization members may try to repress emotions loosened by traumatic events, but it is not possible to imprison them indefinitely. Silence – the inability to speak publicly the truth of one's experience – in organizations is corrosive. It creates cultures of rumor and cover-up. People spend time trying to figure out both the truth and how to disguise it, which takes them away from looking closely at what happened and how to ensure it does not happen again. They cannot learn or heal. The corrosion weakens the system. Inevitably, something bursts, like the sudden torrent of stories of sexual abuse of children by priests spilling out from the Catholic Church. In other organizations there is steady leakage but not yet a bursting, as members are absent or leave altogether because of widespread demoralization, the causes of which are never quite discussed. Organizations slow and finally halt, their members stunned by unexpected disasters like surgical errors or slowly paralyzed by chronic conditions that wear them down emotionally, to the point that they are doing little more than moving in place.

They need not remain that way. Smith and Berg (1987) identify three principles of movement that enable group and organization members to create patterns that get them unstuck. These principles were implicit in the suggestions made in previous chapters of how to function more effectively. They also parallel those that Herman (1997) describes as vital to recovery from trauma.

Move towards anxiety

One principle suggests the importance of moving towards rather than away from the anxiety associated with any event or issue (Smith & Berg 1987). In the Maple Hospital SU, this means that members would have spoken together about the surgical error and its aftermath. This would have occurred in multiple settings, each group convened by its leader, and then the unit as a whole brought together for several sessions. In that process they would have analyzed what occurred, and why, and what to do to ensure it did not occur again, much like the reviews that surgeons in many hospitals routinely conduct after errors. SU members would have expressed their anger, sadness, and guilt. Staff members would inevitably have had to have difficult conversations with one another and address issues that made them anxious, such as the arrogance of surgeons unable to admit that at times they do not remember particular patients; nurses unable to speak up when they believe things are going wrong; and the sense of abandonment and betrayal by hospital administrators who do not support the unit.

Addressing such difficult topics requires supportive group and organizational contexts, and such contexts may be hard to come by, given pulls toward denial and repression in the face of anxiety and painful affect. A certain amount of self-deception is often useful, enabling people to continue working with careseekers who have been abused, have little prospects for meaningful lives, are seriously ill, or dying. Denial and repression aid functional self-deception. However, it can be dysfunctional when preventing people from reflecting on and speaking of the trauma they themselves experience. Trauma researchers refer to the "conspiracy of silence" in describing "no talk" rules that impede people speaking of their trauma to others (Beaton & Murphy 1995). The silencing response presses caregivers to redirect, shut down, minimize or neglect traumatic material (Baranowsky 2002). This may occur in caregivers' relations to careseekers or in their relations with one another. Often enough, it is both.

Traumatized individuals need to tell the stories of their traumas. The narrative includes the events as well as the person's responses and the responses of others (Herman 1997). Facts and emotions must both be expressed. After enough expression and repetitions, the trauma will become less crucial to how people identify their selves (Herman 1997). The individual no longer needs continued efforts at adaptation, completion, and triumph; they no longer feel the compulsion to repeat the trauma in order to master it or the emotions it released. Rather, it can be expressed and thus integrated into daily life. Caregiving organization members whose units are stuck in some fundamental way must also reconstruct their narratives. They must speak of that which haunts them – an event, a series of episodes, or the cumulative assault of their work. They must talk of their experiences and share the emotions they trigger (Frost 2003). In so doing, people can integrate their experiences into their daily work lives and relationships. They will come to some resolution, such that painful events or experiences assume proportionate rather than disproportionate places in their lives. If not, they, like the SU, may be locked within defensive routines that keep alive trauma and its attendant emotions without hope of resolution.

Recognize and reclaim projections

A second principle of movement focuses on group and organization members recognizing how they use others as receptacles of projections in order to define themselves. Splitting and projection, while defending individuals from anxiety, leaves social systems stuck (Smith & Berg 1987). Movement cannot occur unless people are able to explore the full range of their own experiences and emotions. Consider, for example, a marriage in which one partner projects onto the other his need for closeness, and the other, in return, does the same with her need for distance (Scarf 1987). The marriage is stuck within a pattern whereby one partner is constantly seeking more from the other, and is rejected. This pattern enables them, together, to regulate and constrain intimacy within the marriage. However, there can be no movement: the partners, and the marriage itself, will not grow, so long as they cannot, alone and together, explore their own desires for both intimacy and distance.

The same holds true for groups and organizations. When individuals make unrecognized projections they lock one another in roles that constrain movement. In the Maple Hospital SU, unit members split off the angry, vengeful parts of themselves and projected them onto Barbara Nash. Many unit members were angry with the surgeon who had botched the operation and with the arrogance of the surgeons more generally. These members, many of them nurses who thought of themselves as caring and compassionate, implicitly reinforced their nurse manager for treating the surgeons disrespectfully and forcefully. While grumbling about her favoritism, they did not complain so publicly to hospital administrators that her power over the surgeons would be threatened. They were thus able to maintain both the belittling punishment of the surgeons and the image of themselves as compassionate and caring. They could only do this if Barbara Nash acted as a caricature of the angry, demeaning nurse manager.

This sort of process may be understood as a traumatic reaction at the unit level. Trauma disrupts people's relations with others (Herman 1997). Individuals who have been traumatized turn away from most others, their basic sense of trust violated. They heal when they are able to restore that trust through meaningful attachments. In the context of those relationships, survivors integrate the range of their reactions – guilt, anger, sadness, and the like – and come to an understanding of their complete experiences. Similarly, when a unit is traumatized, episodically or cumulatively, members' sense of basic trust is violated. Members cannot easily hold onto all parts of their emotional experiences – hope, anger, disappointment, sadness, and guilt – and thus cast one another into roles that enable those dimensions to exist within the unit as a whole. The unit thus fractures. The unit as a whole cannot then absorb the traumatic experience and integrate its different dimensions. It casts members into specific roles, thereby locking underlying traumas in place.

Groups have more capacity to bear and integrate traumatic experience than individuals (Herman 1997). This suggests a change process for the SU. In the context of gathering together to examine their experiences as a unit, SU members will need to admit the stories that they privately tell themselves. They will need to tell of the characters they assign to one another. It is only by acknowledging, for example, that the nurse manager is perceived as cruel, the surgeons as coldly arrogant, and the nurses as ineffectual that unit members can acknowledge the limits of those characterizations and how they obscure more complicated realities. When unit members are helped – by leaders, consultants, or one another – to see their characterizations of others as *projections* of split-off parts of themselves, insight and change may occur. This will require a series of meetings convened for precisely this purpose.

Leaders facilitate explorations

A third principle of movement focuses on the role of leaders as facilitators of people's explorations of underlying tensions, issues, and events. Reclaiming split-off emotions and reactions is a difficult process. It requires safety, basic trust, and support (Smith & Berg 1987). It requires leadership. Maple Hospital's SU clearly lacked such leadership in the months and years following the surgical event. The then hospital administration CEO, chief of surgery, and nurse manager were all unable or unwilling to convene SU members and facilitate their reflections on the event and its aftermath. Nor did the successive leaders help SU members examine the disturbances in their unit – the relations between surgeons and nurses, the cliques and favoritism, the divisive nurse manager – that arose from the traumatic incident.

In working through trauma, the role of the leader is akin to that of an attachment figure: a trustworthy, secure base on whom others can rely. This role is made complicated by the fact that leaders must be attachment figures for units, not simply for individuals within them. The distinction is crucial. Barbara Nash may well have been a useful leader for nurses she favored. They may have come to her for support, advice and problem-solving. She did not, however, serve the unit as a whole in such ways. She focused on problematic individuals (e.g., offending surgeons, nurses out of favor) rather than on the group's problems with communication, cliques, and a culture of disrespect. She failed to help unit members meet regularly in groups to talk about the traumatic event, and moreover, approach it in terms of the unit's problems, not individuals' problems (see Catherall 1995). It was thus incumbent upon the new chief of surgery and nurse manager to interrupt the isolation and conflict within the unit. They began the process by removing Barbara Nash. They needed to continue by regularly convening unit members and adopting a leadership stance that emphasized listening to, absorbing, digesting, and reacting to members' experiences.

When leaders serve as attachment figures for their units they are more likely to create the conditions of safety necessary for trauma victims to reconstruct their story and restore connections to their communities (Frost 2003). Often enough it is therapists who serve this role for trauma victims. Good therapists bear witness to what occurred, foster insight and empathic connections, and work with the transference and counter-transference within healing relationships (Herman 1997). This offers a model of sorts for leaders in caregiving organizations whose members are stuck in ineffective patterns. While not therapists *per se*, these leaders similarly need to help excavate and bear witness to that which troubles unit members beneath the surface of their work lives. To not do so exacerbates the trauma itself: it is an ongoing betrayal by those in authority that continues to disrupt members' sense of basic trust (Shay 1994).

Letting go, moving on

The Maple Hospital SU's avoidance of its unwanted emotional life came at great cost. The SU sustained five years of anger, blame, and resentment. Relationships were damaged and casualties were created. Some of those who left, like Barbara Nash, did so angrily and bitterly. They were filled like containers from the unit's underlying spring of anger and sadness, and sent away. Some quite probably carried those emotions with them into their new lives, like untreated trauma victims. They bore a disproportionate share of the costs of the unit's social defenses. They sustained personal damage because there was no place for the unit as a whole to talk about the damage to them all.

Processes like this occur in many caregiving organizations: those that have particular traumatic events to which they can point, or more routinely, those that have chronic exposure to traumatic stress that accumulates across months and years of working with careseekers. Their dynamics play out in different ways, but inevitably they are revealed through the stuck patterns in which organization members are trapped as they go about their work. With enough attention, these patterns may be understood as the artifacts of untreated trauma. Traumas occur as a matter of course in caregiving organizations. If they are acknowledged as such, then members may move through the process of resolving them – through narrative, witnessing, and insight. If they are not acknowledged they are unceremoniously buried. Events occur and without public comment sink beneath the surface of organizational life.

Unacknowledged trauma in caregiving organizations means that people cannot fully mourn. Trauma brings loss: of basic trust, of attachments, of identity, of illusions of immortality, of relationships. Loss must be grieved. Explicit grieving allows people their full range of expressions in relation to that which they lost. They come to terms with that loss, placing it within some appropriate context, and can move on. At that point, the story becomes another memory, one without the capacity to cause so much pain; survivors come to identify their selves as more than simply trauma victims (Herman 1997). When grief remains incomplete, trauma continues to attract energy. People cannot move away from it: they are held there by their sense of incompleteness. Unresolved or incomplete mourning traps people in the traumatic process. In such instances people and their units are unable or unwilling to let go of that which wounded them. They cannot move from that place to another.

Part 3

Leading caregiving organizations

The preceding chapters indicate that the nature of caregiving organizations is fundamentally shaped by their members' struggles to work well at multiple levels simultaneously. On one level, there is the technical work of meeting the needs of careseekers. Teachers must offer instruction to students in ways that enable them to learn. Nurses, physicians, and other medical personnel must diagnose and treat patients according to the contours of their specific ailments. Social workers and residential care workers must help their clients navigate the various institutions instrumental in their care and treatment. Clergy must offer sermons, pastoral counseling, and programs that help their congregants with their spiritual and religious questions and needs. Each of these tasks demands a certain technical competence. At another level, there is the work of forming meaningful connections with careseekers who may experience any combination of powerful emotions – fear, anger, joy, excitement, nervousness, sadness, terror – as they attempt to heal, grow, or learn. Such emotions often present as some form of anxiety. Caregiving organization members must manage such emotions and anxiety as they go about the technical work of providing care.

Leaders must also work at both technical and emotional levels in relation to their organization members. Effective leaders understand, intuitively if not explicitly, how closely intertwined are the technical and relational aspects of their members' work lives. They understand that beneath observable daily work and interactions flows an undercurrent of emotions, imported and triggered by careseekers, felt by caregivers and other organization members. If that undercurrent is not acknowledged and understood as such, system-level disturbances are created and maintained. Both the technical and relational aspects of an organization or unit become twisted in some fashion, with disrupting implications for both organization members and those who seek their help.

This complicates the leader's role in caregiving organizations. The leader must do the typical work of leading – creating vision, motivating and engaging others in its clarification and implementation, aligning systems to support visions, and developing others' leadership capacities. Yet there is an additional layer of work as well. The leader must attend to the underlying emotional currents that move beneath the surface. These often present themselves as disturbances, small or large disruptions in how members work or relate. Effective leaders attend carefully to such disturbances. They trace them to their sources. They use them as opportunities to call their members' attention to how well or badly they are accomplishing their primary tasks. They seek to understand and interrupt disturbing patterns, aware that if they did not, the emotional currents will grow stronger and more insistent. They understand, finally, that it is only by attending explicitly to the underlying currents that they can help others become, individually and collectively, resilient.

Leaders in caregiving organizations thus require certain stances and capacities. Part 3 describes these requirements. Chapter 11 clarifies the conditions that leaders need to establish and patrol – the setting of primary tasks, roles, and boundaries – that enable members to engage effectively with one another. Chapter 12 focuses on the leader's need to negotiate the difficult terms of dependency in their relations with organization members. Chapter 13 examines the leader's role as change agent, pressing the organization toward a collective maturity. Together, these chapters sketch a portrait of leaders who are able and willing to develop their own and others' capacities to work effectively in emotionally complex environments.

Chapter 11

The leadership task

The leadership of caregiving organizations is both like and unlike that of other organizations. There remain the constants of leadership: creating vision and mission; establishing goals and objectives, and enabling systems and structures; motivating, challenging, empowering, and inspiring others; providing resources; and aligning people's efforts with one another and with the environments in which they work, using reward, information management, and hierarchical systems (Kouzes & Posner 2002). Leaders across a variety of organizations and industries must perform some variation of these behaviors if their organizations are to thrive. In caregiving organizations, leaders must, in addition, enable resilience throughout their organizations, and maintain real systems of caregiving. Caregiving leaders who ably perform the classic leadership behaviors, but who cannot help members remain resilient in the face of inevitable stress and anxiety, sow the seeds of caregiving system breakdowns. They do so in spite of their best intentions otherwise.

Resilience in social systems is a product of the collective. Individuals vary in how resilient they are but it is their collective resilience that is of concern to effective leaders. Collective resilience develops only when caregiving organization members join together in meaningful ways: to share information, solve problems, make sense of their experiences, and provide support. People create bridges that mark system-level resilience when they routinely come together in such ways and integrate organizational divisions. When they routinely traverse those bridges in search of collaboration and support they create working relationships that sustain them during times of stress and anxiety. It is in the collective that resilience is sustained past the turnover of individual members.

What caregiving organizations and their members need is not simply technical, strategic leadership. Effective leaders do not simply develop strategy and point others toward implementation. Nor do they only manage finances, develop revenue streams, and create programs. They enable group and organizational members to join together to reflect upon their experiences in their roles, express rather than act out or defend against strong emotion and anxiety, and develop productive mechanisms by which to effectively withstand that which assaults them in the daily course of their work with careseekers. They focus on shoring up the resilience of organizations and their members. They do so in two ways. First, they help create the conditions necessary for members to engage one another in non-superficial ways. These conditions include specifying clear primary tasks, delineating appropriate roles and authority, and managing appropriate organizational boundaries. Second, they help convene people in various forums or settings that promote resilience. These two leadership functions are discussed in this chapter and illustrated using material drawn from the case studies in Part 2.

Creating conditions for engagement

Resilience is created when individuals absorb, express, reflect on, and learn from their emotions at work. Since this process in organizational life is largely social – people joining with others to make sense of their collective experiences – individuals require a sense of safety to engage this sequence (Kahn 1992). Safety allows people to be vulnerable and take risks in openly exploring emotions and anxieties. People must be willing to engage *themselves*, as it were, when engaging with others to figure out their deeper experiences of caregiving work.

These engagements occur in the context of various forums: supervisions, teams, group and department meetings, management meetings. Caregiving organization members will not be able to engage in such forums, however, unless three basic conditions exist at work: clear primary tasks; appropriate roles and authority; and appropriate organizational boundaries. These conditions define resilient cultures, and mirror those required for the construction of holding environments (Shapiro & Carr 1991). When such conditions are *not* met, members are moved to disengage, invoking defensive routines of which they are often unaware. When these conditions *are* met, members are more likely to engage the difficult work of examining the emotional undercurrents that threaten to render them ineffective. The leadership task thus involves first creating the basic conditions for engagement.

Clarifying primary tasks

The primary tasks of caregiving organizations can prove quite elusive. While they can often be articulated reasonably well – a school's primary task is to educate all students to the best of their abilities, a treatment center's primary task is to promote patients' emotional and physical growth and independence – they just as often get lost in practice (Lyth 1988). Emotionally and psychologically easier tasks may subsume them. The cases in Part 2 showed how various social defenses gained currency and power because they offered members the chance to withdraw from primary tasks and move toward some substituted reality that caused less, or at least more tolerable, anxiety.

Leaders thus need to monitor primary tasks. They must consistently examine the extent to which members' efforts are on-task or off-task. They must attend to what members do, not simply what they say they do; it is within patterns of individual, group, and intergroup behavior that the actual tasks that people are working on are revealed. Leaders must also examine how they themselves may collude with the loss of task. On-task leadership requires leaders to constantly scrutinize what they and others do in the light of primary tasks. Leaders who do not do so are in danger of abusing their power, of serving their own needs at the expense of those of others (Obholzer 1994). Their own needs, in this case, might well involve the desire to avoid the difficult emotions and anxieties moving toward them, like a steadily mounting wall of water, should they hold others to their primary tasks. This is not so much an abuse of power as its abdication. Leaders may abdicate entirely their responsibility to point members toward their primary tasks, unwilling themselves to deal with members' reactions to being held to those tasks.

At Greenvale Residential Treatment Center (Chapter 7), organizational and departmental leaders were unwilling to monitor the primary task, resulting in the loss of that task by staff members. They did not examine relations within and across the residential, educational, and clinical departments in the light of the need to constantly integrate clients' experiences and create a therapeutic milieu. Nor did they hold staff accountable for behaviors that undermined such integration. Instead, they allowed the agency to create a series of diversions – turf battles, personality conflicts, and the like – that drew attention away from concerted efforts toward the difficult task of integrating clients' experiences.

Monitoring the primary task at Greenvale would have required leaders to regularly articulate and reinforce a model of integration (the therapeutic milieu) and train staff members to enact it in daily practice. They would have also needed to help staff members accept the limitations of that model in practice. Obholzer (1994: 174) suggests that caregivers need help in accepting their own powerlessness: the limitations of what they might reasonably do. He writes: "A great deal of what goes on is not about dramatic rescue but about having to accept one's relative powerlessness in the presence of pain, decrepitude and death. Staff members are ill prepared for this in their training, and in their work practice there is often no socially sanctioned outlet for their distress."

As part of staff training, Greenvale leaders would thus have needed to teach staff about the reasonable limits to what the agency might reasonably accomplish with abused, disturbed adolescents who had little capacity for trust, attachment, and intimacy. Leaders and members alike would have had to come to terms with the limitations of their own power to dramatically intervene and rescue their clients, while still retaining hope on behalf of those clients. To the extent that Greenvale leaders were unable to do this, they remained invested in the diversions staged by the staff.

Delineating roles and authority

Primary tasks are best served when organization members assume given roles appropriately (Shapiro & Carr 1991). Social defenses flourish when people assume roles that help them manage anxieties rather than engage work. Department heads assume the roles of warrior chiefs, defending their turfs. Nurses assume policing roles, warily inspecting surgeons. Supervisors assume roles in which they are protected and cared for by social workers, who in turn take on nurturing roles that leave them unprotected. Each of these scenarios represents the loss of roles that best serve primary tasks. Each represents a subversion – the loss, inversion, or bloating – of members' appropriate authority. Each maintains a social defense that creates casualties – of organization members and careseekers. Each occurs with leaders' unspoken collusions.

Effective caregiving organization leaders attend closely to how members enact their roles and assume authority. Appropriate roles are those that afford members opportunities to contribute to primary tasks in concert with others. Appropriate authority is that which allows members to assume responsibility and ownership commensurate with their institutional roles. The leader continuously monitors the extent to which they and organization members are enacting roles that are on-task and vested with neither too much nor too little authority in the institution. When members occupy roles that are off-task, and defensive in nature, they are less available for on-task work. They are less accessible – emotionally, cognitively, physically – to careseekers and to one another. They are less engaged.

At Project Home (Chapter 5), the social workers occupied two roles – as protectors of their supervisor, and as abandoned children within the agency – that had little to do with the primary task of caring for their clients. Neither of those roles enabled them meaningful opportunities to participate and contribute in the agency, since those roles depended on their relative isolation from agency leaders and administrators. Similarly, the supervisor's role – the needy, overwhelmed maternal figure – left her unable to contribute to the agency's primary task and without the authority to protect the social workers. The agency's director colluded with members assuming inappropriate, covert roles and too little authority; more generally, he colluded with the social defense system that created casualties among the social workers and left him and the other administrators relatively protected from anxiety.

A more effective agency director would attend more closely to what the social workers actually did in the agency. He would, like a detective following clues, look for the pattern beneath a set of data: the inverted relationship between social workers and their supervisor, the social workers' isolation within the agency, their ongoing turnover. That trail would quite reasonably have led to the conclusion that the social workers were not able to form the stable attachments with their clients necessary to guide clients toward their own stable attachments with families and communities. Rather than blaming the social workers for their failings, the director would have examined why the agency was unable to hold onto them. The director would have had to look closely at his own collusion: his own abandoning of the social workers, his failures to manage the supervisor, the gulf that he promoted between social workers and administrators. This can only occur, of course, when such leaders care more for their clients than for their own needs to avoid anxiety or understand their own human failings.

Managing organizational boundaries

The leader is also responsible for creating and maintaining appropriate boundaries. Appropriate boundaries are those that are neither too permeable nor too impermeable (Alderfer 1980a), enabling people to access information and resources but not leaving them overly exposed to their environments. The various social defenses described in earlier chapters were marked by the loss of boundaries. Boundaries between units were drawn so tightly that organizations split into warring regions, unable to work together on behalf of care-seekers. Or, they were drawn so loosely that units all but disappeared, their members unable to identify and work effectively with one another. Members and leaders alike use such inappropriate boundaries to reinforce the loss of task, role, and authority that mark flights from anxiety.

The leader's role in maintaining appropriate boundaries includes protecting members from external disturbance. Disturbances occur when transactions across unit boundaries distract members from their primary tasks. These might include, for example, upsetting rumors or stereotypes that flood an organization. Or they may involve a set of workflow processes – the transferring of patients from one hospital unit to another, or the investigation of restraints in a residential treatment center – that cause friction. Leaders must manage boundaries to minimize such disturbances (Miller 1993) and they often do so by maintaining positions on work group boundaries that enable them to effectively bridge and manage transactions between units and environments (Bayes & Newton 1985).

The Sudbury Hospital ER (Chapter 8) lacked such boundary management. Patients overran the ER. When patients were ready to be admitted to another hospital unit, relations between the units prevented this from occurring. The medical director was unable to either create more effective relations with his counterparts in other units or work effectively with hospital administration to enable such integration. He routinely created disturbances within the unit himself by repeating rumors, openly feuding with other administrators, and undermining physicians in front of nurses. He could not manage the boundaries within the unit itself, between senior and junior nurses and between nurses and physicians. He left the unit divided, stirred up, and overwhelmed.

A more effective ER leader would have worked with hospital administration to convene the relevant unit directors and develop a strategy for relieving some of the pressure on the ER. This would also have meant working with the administration to increase the resources – patient beds, nursing personnel, and equipment – necessary to fully staff the unit and serve the increasing number of patients flooding in. Finally, a more effective leader would have tried to create bridges between the different informal divisions and cliques that had suffused the unit, filling the vacuum left by the lack of emphasis on collective goals and purposes. Such bridging involves first communicating the unit's primary task, and second, putting forth the vision of how members need to work together across formal and informal boundaries to achieve that task. A more effective medical director, in other words, would define leadership partly in terms of boundary management.

Convening for resilience

When primary tasks, roles and authority, and boundaries are appropriately clear and managed, it becomes possible for caregiving organization members to create resilient work relationships. Effective leaders convene various forums or settings for that purpose. Department heads convene teachers, supervisors convene social workers, and nurse managers convene nurses to surface issues, share experiences and join together in the face of anxiety generated by their work with clients and patients. Middle managers convene cross-functional groups of unit leaders to raise and resolve issues concerning front-line caregivers. Senior managers convene middle managers to integrate their efforts to solve such issues. Executive directors, principals, super-intendents, and other senior leaders convene others to share and solve problems affecting their organizations. At each level, effective leaders provide purposes, settings, resources, and boundaries. They hold fast to the process of enabling others to surface and work through issues without hijacking that process.

Convening refers to the gathering together of others who join forces in the service of a primary task. Such joining has a number of purposes. The most obvious is the performance of the work itself. People meet to develop plans and strategies for their work projects and processes, share information and resources, solve problems together, and generally depend on one another in the course of their work together. Effective leaders in caregiving organiza-tions, however, convene members for more complicated purposes as well. They strive to create, in Main's (1995) phrase, "cultures of inquiry" that enable system-level resilience to be created and maintained.

Hinshelwood (2001: 112) offers an extensive analysis of cultures of inquiry. He describes them as "cultures consciously aimed at questioning and reflect-ing on why we do things like this." Such cultures emerge when reflective spaces are opened and maintained. These spaces might occur in supervision, in staff meetings, in administrative sessions. In such contexts, workers inquire into patterns of behavior. They examine and respect reality rather than engage in wishful thinking or denial. They are supportive and non-judgmental. They remain curious rather than defensive. They reflect together. "In healthy action," writes Hinshelwood (2001: 101), "reflection intervenes between experiences and ensuing action." Without such reflective spaces, caregiving organization members routinely sink into defensive or other dysfunctional patterns of behavior.

Cultures of inquiry are marked by people working with the raw materials of their emotional experiences to inform their work. People put out to one another their actual experiences (what happened) and their emotional reactions (what they felt during and about what happened). They express anger, resentment, longing, fear, sadness, or whatever else they feel or felt. This emotional material offers valuable information about what is occurring within the social system. This mirrors the psychoanalytic premise of the existence and value of transference and counter-transference. The sharing of emotions also creates what Hinshelwood (2001: 178) refers to as the "linking-up" of system members: they become linked through exchanging and interpreting emotions.

This linking, a joining together in the face of strong emotional experiences, forms the foundation for resilience. Once shared and accepted as valid by a group, emotions become the province of the collective. They are taken in and dispersed, such that no one member must hold onto and be potentially disabled by them. Hinshelwood (2001: 139) describes this as a "relationship network that accepts anxiety and distress, and can contain it, through reflection, by giving it meaning." Resilience is created and enacted through absorption – of emotion, distress, anxiety – by relationship networks whose containing capacities are stronger than those of individual members themselves. This is the logic of the culture of inquiry, and of resilient caregiving systems more generally: sharing and dispersing the inevitable distress renders it less powerful. "The practice of constant enquiry," notes Hinshelwood (2001: 113) "is the basis of the survival of an alive and healthy institution." It is what enables workers to "confront together the projection and introjection systems and to help rescue one another when one or more of them are caught" (Lyth 1988: 248).

Effective leaders ensure that such inquiry is woven into caregiving organization structures and processes. This is no easy task. "A fight has to go on to keep open a space in the working day, but more importantly, a space within the minds of the professionals, a space where questioning can survive" (Hinshelwood 2001: 113). The effective leader continuously wages that fight. He or she enables members to have ongoing places to reflect on what is happening to them, thus lessening their need to act out and defend against painful experiences. He or she struggles to enable members to be what Schön (1983) termed "reflective practitioners."

Leaders may convene members in different settings. Each setting is marked by particular characteristics with which leaders and members must contend in order to render it useful for creating resilience.

Supervision

Supervision, as discussed in Chapter 3, is one setting in which people may receive interpretation and support. Supervision offers the chance for caregivers to reflect on their practices with careseekers. It also offers the opportunity for supervisors to relieve anxiety (through its expression) and to learn something of value about the institution (through projective identification). Supervision is understood partly as an emotional exchange system, through which issues move from careseeker to staff to supervisor. As Hinshelwood (2001: 140) describes, "The supervisor's role is to be a setting that can in some way take the anxiety and do some thinking about it. This is the creation of a reflective space, the purpose of which is to convert something anxious into something communicated. Then that something, reflected upon and now more meaningful, can be passed back down the chain."

The effective supervisor thus absorbs, digests, and provides for supervisees in the way that caregivers work with careseekers, as described in Chapter 1. In supervision the aim is to enhance staff members' capacities for resilience: showing them that their distress may be contained, made sense of, and made useful for their work with others. Supervisors may engage this process with groups as well as individuals. Group supervision enables relationship networks to be created, whose members can learn together to bear painful affect.

The supervisor at Project Home (Chapter 5) failed to enable the resilience of the agency's social workers: she maintained an emotional distance from the social workers: she met with and listened to them, but she did not absorb them to the point that they experienced her empathy and understanding. They in turn learned not to present her with material that would require her empathy. They did this in part to protect her, sensing her fragility, and in part to protect themselves from the disappointment of asking for and not receiving help. The roles of supervisor and supervisee were thus abandoned, the task of supervision lost. A more effective process would begin with the supervisor's repeated demonstration of her capacity to take in, absorb, and re-present the social workers' experiences in ways that leave them feeling empathized with and with more insight into their work with clients. This would engage a cycle whereby the social workers increasingly learn to interpret their own experiences, which they check with the supervisor, who helps them tackle ever more complex dynamics. Such cycles enable resilience.

Staff meetings

Staff meetings enable department members to raise issues, develop shared understandings of experiences and events, and agree to consistent work practices. They offer another type of opportunity as well: the creation of meaningful attachments. When department members are able to speak of their actual experiences of their work and interactions, in the service of making that work better, they form attachments that, over time, translate into the relationship networks underlying cultures of inquiry. Members can absorb the distress that enters the department, disperse it among themselves, and work with rather than be disabled by it.

The department head is an instrumental part of this process. It is the leader's job to structure and manage staff meetings such that the distress is expressed, worked with by the unit, and converted into useful insights and support. In practice this means that leaders regularly make room for department members to talk about their work experiences – stressful situations, emotional highs and lows, nagging concerns, and the like – and help them examine those experiences for what they might reveal about the unit's work more generally. Leaders need to ensure that members feel they can speak candidly of their experiences and emotions without risk of isolation or scapegoating, i.e., without being the object of others' defensive moves away from anxiety. Effective department heads monitor the process by which members share, absorb, and make sense of their experiences, such that no member is left holding anxiety inappropriately.

Effective department leaders take seriously the idea that units have emotional lives that must be publicly excavated and tended to. The medical director of the Sudbury Hospital ER (Chapter 8) did not understand this principle. The ER was split into various groupings that fractured the unit in ways destructive to the task of tending to an enormous patient flow. The medical director colluded by allowing the groupings to exist unimpeded. Indeed, he contributed to the divisions by meeting regularly only with his physician colleagues. A more effective department head would frame the leadership task partly in terms of breaking down the overly rigid boundaries between the formal (nurses/physicians) and informal (new/old nurses) groups, to allow for the flow of information and support across the department as a whole. In practice this would mean regular staff meetings with all department members, in which time and space were made available for ER members to talk about their frustrations, concerns, ideas, enthusiasms, and work with patients and one another. Over time, led correctly, staff meetings can become regular places for department members to join together in the face of stress.

Task forces

Caregiving organizations also utilize task forces, quality circles, and other types of temporary committee to look into particularly important or troubling issues. Such issues – medical errors in hospitals, low scores on standardized tests in high schools, increasing use of restraints in residential treatment centers, increasing dropout rates in alcohol treatment facilities, and the like – often cut across organizations. They require the representation of different functions, departments, hierarchical levels, and other organizational groups. Task forces present significant opportunities to build bridges between those groups. When group representatives form attachments with one another they are able to create better flows of information, engage in problem-solving, and stake out common ground on behalf of integrating their respective groups. Meaningful attachments also translate over time into relationship networks capable of absorbing and interpreting distress imported by task force representatives.

The role of the task force leader is particularly crucial here. Leaders not only delineate goals and objectives, processes, sub-groups, and timetables for task forces, they also help members transmit, absorb, interpret, and integrate emotional material. They do this by emphasizing how the task force is a useful microcosm of the organization. They help task force members examine how their words and behaviors inevitably represent the experiences, attitudes, emotions, and perspectives of their groups. By examining what gets presented during the team's work, leaders and task force members can begin to interpret and understand the relations between the groups, and from there, how the organization more generally has been dealing with (and often defending against) its core issues.

The task force leader thus makes time and space for members to express and interpret their experiences. Without such expression task force representatives (and by extension, their groups) remain divided in unexamined ways. The task force at Thurston High School (Chapter 9) sought to create a new program enabling students to form relationship networks with staff and one another. The task force was a microcosm of the school, containing representatives of gender, racial, seniority, and hierarchical groups. The vice-principal led the committee. The committee was paralyzed by its unaddressed differences, particularly around race, and members spent much of their time ignoring or battling with one another. Such paralysis would have been reduced had the vice-principal pressed members to express what they really thought and felt – their hopes and fears, their perceptions of their own and others' groups – and tried to interpret and understand that material in terms of what it meant for the program and the school. If the vice-principal had been able to maintain that focus he and the committee members would have learned a great deal about how to structure a program aimed at enabling students and staff to speak openly with one another. An intervention in the committee itself would have helped interrupt dysfunctional patterns in the school more generally.

Management teams

Management teams offer another vehicle for integration. They function best when they are framed as teams rather than groups, i.e., when their tasks are at least partly collective. Like athletes in a team sport, managers must work together to achieve a measurable, team-level outcome, to which their individual performances directly contribute. Treated and led as such, management teams enable senior executives to integrate differentiated units. They offer the opportunity for middle- or senior-level managers to share information, solve common problems, develop strategy and its implementation, and more generally provide their own leaders with an integrated portrait of the larger organization.

Management teams contain people who operate at the boundaries of their units. Heads of departments, functional areas, programs, and other divisions occupy roles that require them to be both inside and outside their units. They must connect enough with unit members to guide and support their work. They must also connect with other managers as they traverse their organizations to procure resources, develop strategy, and pursue projects that demand collaborative efforts. Such "boundary spanners," as discussed in Chapter 7, are susceptible to being loaded up with projections. Members of departments, units, programs, or functional areas may project upon the most visible members of other areas (the formal heads) those characteristics which they associate with those other areas. Such projections serve defensive purposes, often enough, and make it difficult for leaders to engage clearly with one another. Projections about area leaders tend to lock in place prevailing social defenses and it becomes difficult for managers to perceive one another in ways that contradict those defenses.

Effective executives use management teams not simply to accomplish work or help develop and implement strategy but to learn about relations between areas and divisions. They accept that management teams, like task forces, consist of group representatives who have absorbed the perspectives, emotions, and beliefs of their constituencies. They look to see how that material plays itself out within the management team itself. They understand that relations between various areas represented on the management team will reveal themselves in the interactions among team members. They look to assess those relations and help their managers develop corresponding insights and understandings.

This did not occur at the Greenvale Residential Treatment Center (Chapter 7). The executive director and other members of the administration met regularly with the three department heads. Relations between the three heads were in constant disrepair. They battled publicly, spread rumors about each other, and encouraged their department members to act territorially. The senior administrators framed the department heads' behavior as inappropriate, and blamed their difficult personalities. They were unwilling to hold them accountable, colluding with the distraction that battling provided. Ideally, the senior administrators would have interpreted, and enabled the department heads to interpret as well, the struggles for what they represented about the agency as a whole. The battles and role confusions between the department heads reflected the absence, in practice, of an integrated therapeutic model that honored the contributions of the residential, clinical, and educational components necessary to help the clients. The dysfunctional relations between the department heads reflected that absence and needed to be understood as a plea for support and insight.

Large-scale meetings

Large-scale meetings, such as divisional or organizational retreats, offer opportunities for members to create attachments with one another that transcend the boundaries that typically separate them. There are various purposes for such gatherings. They can be vehicles by which new leadership, strategies, programs, and organizational changes are developed, announced or worked with in some fashion. They can enable people to share information that typically remains locked within disparate units. They can address shared problems. They can celebrate achievements. They can be opportunities for organization members to gain perspective on their collective work and make decisions about future directions. In caregiving organizations they can also enable members to develop larger relationship networks similar to those created in supervisory relations and departments. These larger networks enable people to understand how their experiences at work are related to one another and to the task of their organizations.

In large-scale meetings, people can develop insight into how their work experiences are shaped by the larger system of which they are a part. This only occurs when those who convene these meetings are able to guide people toward such insight. Senior executives must create settings in which people feel safe enough to risk making their real thoughts and feelings known. This requires leaders to model the way – to take the lead in making the undiscussable discussable. Organization members need to know that it is acceptable, even required, for them to speak the open secrets that infiltrate their organizations. For example, frustration and anger with clients and with those who seemingly coddle or are too harsh with them; sadness about increasingly sick patients whose bodies do not respond to new medications; anger and confusion about a rash of medication errors committed by poorly-trained nurses; longings for administration to walk the floors and resentment of their seeming abandonment of the unit. There are many such open secrets in caregiving organizations. When they are expressed, members can join together for insight and support. When they are not expressed, the secrets contribute to people's disengagements from one another.

Consider, for example, the rage, sadness, and frustration that marked the Maple Hospital SU (Chapter 10). These emotions were triggered by a surgical error. The error became an open secret within the unit and within the hospital more generally. Neither the chief of surgery nor the nurse manager called unit members together. If they had, several purposes might have been accomplished. At a practical level, people could have received the same information about the event rather than try and sift through multiple rumors. They could have examined the event and its contributing factors, and learned how to prevent such errors in the future. At an emotional level, people could have expressed their feelings and thus have less reason to defend against them by splintering into warring factions. They could have developed relationship networks that would have absorbed and dispersed the distress emanating from the event and its aftermath. Neither the unit leaders nor the hospital administrators convened the members. They left them to their own coping strategies, which seemingly protected some staff members but undermined their resilience as a unit.

Holding the fort

The leadership task, then, is twofold. Leaders establish the conditions – clear tasks, roles, authority, and boundaries – that enable caregiving organization members to safely join together in expressive rather than defensive relationships. They also convene members, bringing them together in various contexts that, over time, ignite the relationship networks through which system-level resilience is created and maintained. It is only through such networks that the anxiety, distress and other emotions infiltrating caregiving organizations are appropriately dispersed and borne.

The leader faces significant pulls to move away from this task. The social defenses that spring up to ward off anxiety are themselves quite resilient. People form habits of thought and action with which they try to protect themselves from experiencing anxiety. Those protective habits may enable them to ignore or withstand distress, but often at the expense of others' abilities to do so. Anxiety, anger, or sadness get pushed over to another team member, or sub-group, or department; they in turn get overloaded and cannot remain resilient in the face of distress. Leaders may collude with these processes. Indeed, they have the power to ensure that less powerful others contain the distress, such that they do not have to. The case studies presented earlier are replete with examples of precisely this. They reveal social workers, junior nurses, childcare workers, and other front-line caregivers absorbing disproportionate amounts of anxiety and other disturbing emotions that affect their leaders and senior administrators relatively little. Effective leaders, conversely, are careful about how their own habits of thought and action leave them in danger of colluding with social defenses against anxiety.

The effective leader must thus hold tightly to the task of creating resilience. He or she must hold the fort, as it were. In part, this means withstanding members' assaults as they retreat to defensive routines. Leaders have several recourses here. First, they can maintain a clear-eyed, insistent focus on interpreting the patterns of behavior within and between groups. These patterns provide clues as to whether people and their groups are on- or off-task. Effective leaders consistently examine others' behaviors, questioning whether they are in the service of meeting careseeker's needs. They speak directly of what they find. They encourage others to do similarly. They are diagnosticians. They are so invested in the primary tasks, and use them to ground their actions so consistently, that they offer a solid foundation on which others can depend as they too bring themselves closer to those tasks.

Second, leaders can insist on the use of regular forums for members to reflect upon their experiences and practices. Effective leaders help others withstand pressures to push away reflection. Such pressures derive partly from the hectic pace of organizational life. Organization members are always in action and reaction, and they pause little for reflection. This serves social defenses, of course, which can only be interrupted when they are reflected upon and understood as such. The manic pace with which many members work is partly an avoidance of such interruptions; it is an avoidance of the emotions that might well flood people if they created space for that to occur. Effective leaders press for such interruptions. They press subordinates to devote regular time for reflection, they understand that these interruptions will temporarily destabilize people as they struggle with what lies beneath their unquestioned habits. But they know too that the alternative is more destructive: primary tasks get lost, and with them the welfare of both careseekers and those who serve them.

Third, leaders can get some outside help. It is difficult for leaders, by themselves, to diagnose and interrupt dysfunctional patterns of behavior. A fair amount of the work referenced here – Jacques (1974), Lyth (1988), Miller (1993), Obholzer and Roberts (1994), Rice (1963), Shapiro and Carr (1991) and others working in the tradition of the Tavistock Institute – reflects the premise that external consultation offers a valuable resource for organizational change, particularly that requiring a loosening of the grip of social defenses. Effective consultation enables organization members to look closely at their patterns, moved by curiosity and concern for careseekers and themselves. Good consultants, like good therapists, hold leaders and members alike to the task of examining the choices that they make and their ensuing consequences, and support them in developing increasingly functional patterns of thought and behavior. Effective leaders allow themselves, and not incidentally, their members, to be helped in such ways.

Engaging these steps is difficult work. Leaders will need to interrupt the press in organizations toward action. Many organizations whose members face daily anxiety develop cultures of action, characterized by a manic pace of work, an emphasis on overly demanding or ambitious deadlines, rushed decision-making in the face of incomplete information, and seemingly constant changes in organizational structures and systems. While each of these is seemingly defensible, given the amount and pace of information in modern organizational life, together they create a culture in which organization members are pressed to act rather than reflect. Effective leaders interrupt these cultures in small, meaningful ways by modeling the act of pausing and reflecting at crucial junctures. They do this even as they themselves feel the press to make decisions, take action, produce. They understand that action without reflection may be a reaction to anxiety, a way to fight or flee from the experience of impotence. They also understand that organizational norms, such as those dictating how meetings are run or how decisions are vetted, may either collude with or alter such anxious reactions.

Chapter 12

Negotiating dependency

Leaders make decisions. They react to information. They defer to others or are quite directive. They manage others' anxieties while struggling with their own. They exhort, discipline, comfort, and motivate. They convene and listen to others. How leaders perform such behaviors is a matter of their particular mixtures of temperament, training, comfort, and ability. Some are able to perform some of the acts necessary to lead effectively, such as making decisions, and not others, such as including and engaging others. Some are less able to guide and direct, preferring to let others assume organizational authority. Others quite naturally involve themselves just enough to guide and support others while enabling them to take ownership of their work. Each leader constructs certain relationships with others based on his or her tendencies and abilities. In caregiving organizations, those relationships powerfully shape members' abilities to remain resilient.

Caregiving organization leaders are the linchpins of the systems by which care flows to careseekers. Careseekers bring their needs, anxieties, and desires to teachers, nurses, physicians, childcare workers, clergy, and the like. These caregivers are the focal points for careseekers' needs, their desires for help, ministration, and nurturing. Ideally, caregivers absorb and attempt to learn from careseekers' experiences, the better to teach and care for them. They themselves become filled with careseekers' hopes, fears, desires, and emotions. In the context of supervision and other work relationships, they may release what they have absorbed. Ideally, as noted in Chapter 3, that material is digested by others within the system, made sense of, and offered back to caregivers in the form of insight and support. The system as a whole thus takes in and works with careseekers, with the primary caregivers most directly involved in the actual delivery of care.

In this process leaders become the ultimate attachment figures. When the caregiving system works well – when careseekers are consistently supported and helped in their healing, growing, and learning, and caregivers are left intact and resilient in the process – it is because leaders provide basic levels of security, support, and insight. They establish holding environments in which staff members are able to express, reflect upon, and develop strategies for dealing with problematic situations (Kahn 2001). They display enough curiosity to allow others to feel inquired about rather than interrogated or evaluated. Members go about their work knowing that if they find themselves startled in some fashion – a troubling situation with a client or student, a traumatic event, the sudden emergence of their own anxiety – they can avail themselves of a leader able to calm them, help them develop perspective and insight, turn them back towards their tasks, and support their progress. Caregiving organization members quite naturally look to their leaders to offer such security.

This is not always a calmly-ordered process. Members of caregiving organizations often converge on their leaders. They seek answers. They seek support. They seek help for nameless struggles whose contours they cannot fully articulate. They seek witnesses to their joys and frustrations. They want many things. At their finest, caregiving leaders are able to meet some needs and help staff members enlarge their own capacities to meet still other needs. They create and sustain holding environments for staff members and temporarily contain what others cannot, just as the caregivers do for those for whom they care. This frees staff members up to work on the problems they encounter unencumbered by otherwise paralyzing emotions. It also allows caregiving leaders to model the process by which careseekers ought to be worked with. When leaders are able to create such holding environments, staff members have a visceral experience of what that feels like and are therefore more likely to try and recreate that experience for others.

This last point is crucial. In these organizations, members look to leaders as if they could, and indeed should, solve the knottiest of problems and make the most painful of emotions disappear. This is part wish, of course. Staff members wish for their leaders to be omnipotent, able to heal and resolve at will, like careseekers wish of their caregivers. They thus inspect their leaders quite closely. They look to see if they are up to the task of caring for and supporting them. They look to see if they are strong enough to hold them. They look to see if their leaders' temperaments, agendas, or ambitions will override their stated goals. They look to see what leaders do with their own infallibilities as clues about what they should do with their own. This level of scrutiny can be unnerving for leaders who experience the weight of others' expectations pressing down upon them. Nevertheless, the fact that caregiving organization members pay such attention gives leaders a powerful tool by which to influence others. Leaders can model in their own relations with staff members how they would like staff to relate to one another and to careseekers.

Effective leaders thus contain others' anxiety and model appropriate behaviors in order to help enlarge members' capacities for resilience. Leaders assume various roles in the service of this task. They direct others when necessary. They coach and facilitate, posing problems and helping others reach useful conclusions. They manage boundaries between groups, using their authority to protect people and projects. They are good enough caregivers themselves, ministering appropriately to people who need temporary holding and respite. In these organizations, effective leaders are those who understand that their work includes managing the emotional life running beneath the more observable work life of projects, budgets, and strategy meetings. They function at both levels simultaneously. They take up their positions as both heads of units and of systems of caregiving that ideally underlie those units. To do this, leaders must negotiate the dependence that inevitably pulls upon them.

Pulls toward dependence

The knottiest issue for leaders in caregiving organizations is that of dependency. Caregiving organization members have quite real dependency needs. Their work is emotionally as well as technically and cognitively demanding. They get exhausted and burned out. They encounter situations that pose problems they cannot easily solve. They get overwhelmed by the amount of work they have to do and the people who require their assistance. They need to be able to depend on their leaders and supervisors to help them get respite, gain perspective and insight, feel good about their work, and hold onto their tasks. Leaders must make themselves available to provide such support. Yet when they do, they run the risk of getting overwhelmed themselves with the needs of members that are rooted in irrational longings for dependency that, by definition, cannot be fully met or resolved. An insistent longing for or rage at others for not meeting one's bottomless needs to be taken care of marks irrational dependency. These are powerful pulls, like undercurrents, that threaten the adult functioning of caregiving organization leaders and members alike.

One source of irrational dependency is "parallel process" stemming from the needs and longings of careseekers. The underlying basic assumption of caregiving organizations, as noted in Chapter 6, is that of dependency. Careseekers wish to be cared for – to be healed, taught, comforted, ministered to. They also wish, albeit less consciously, to believe in the omnipotent powers of caregivers. Faith is a powerful part of the healing process (Miller 1993). If only they are perfectly dependent on their caregivers, the unconscious logic of careseekers holds, their needs will be perfectly met. Caregivers also absorb this. Even as they are consciously aware of their own fallibility with careseekers, they too are attracted to the wish that their own leaders will take care of them perfectly. They unconsciously mirror the careseekers and look to their leaders as they themselves are looked at, as people able to meet or frustrate longings.

Such parallel processes often create a prevailing, unconscious assumption that leaders are apart, above, and all-powerful, and their followers less competent and able. This split is rooted in the healthy/unhealthy, helper/helpless, powerful/powerless archetypes that lie beneath the helping professions (Guggenbuhl-Craig 1971). In hospitals, for example, there is great pressure upon staff members to be healthy and powerful, leaving the patients to be ill, obedient, and grateful (Main 1995). Interactions are between the helpful and the helpless. The pull then is for caregivers and careseekers to collude in acting as if the former are all-knowing and the latter helpless, as if such a formula will guarantee the required healing, growing, learning, and ministering. This formula gets transposed into the relations between organization leaders and members, who are pulled toward the same types of unrealistic dependency.

A second pull toward dependency is the implicit relationship between a caregiving organization and the family, as noted in Chapter 2. The primary task of the family is to ensure the continued development of its members (Shapiro & Carr 1991). This involves, at its core, parents and other primary caregivers taking care of children – feeding them, clothing them, ministering to them when they are ill or upset, teaching them social and cognitive skills. When individuals enter caregiving organizations, in whatever role, they carry with them the memory of those family systems and all the needs that were or were not expressed and met. They use their memory to guide their actions, to create familiarity. They unconsciously map relations of authority between caregiver and careseeker, and leader and member, on the basis of parent-child relationships and act accordingly.

Third, some caregivers are more or less susceptible to longing to be cared for perfectly by authority figures. Some caregivers join caregiving organizations *because* of their own unmet needs for nurturing (Dartington 1994). Their unconscious hope is that in the context of their relations with their leaders they will receive the type of unconditional regard and care they had not received fully earlier in their lives. They wish to continue journeys toward healing and learning that had been halted in some fashion. They unconsciously identify, indeed, may over-identify, with the careseekers' journeys. The unmet, often unconscious needs of staff members may thus find expression in their longings for and frustrations with their leaders.

A fourth pull toward irrational dependency relations is social defenses. Caregiving organization members may come to vest a great deal of authority in leaders who come to symbolize, in the way of a talisman or a superstition, protection from harm. An example of this was presented in Chapter 6, when members of an organization that had survived near collapse allowed themselves to be dominated by the leader who acted as their savior. This relation of abject dependence became a cornerstone of the organization's social defense system. Members acted as if the CEO would take care of them in a turbulent environment even as they consciously understood that he cared little for them. They disabled themselves in return for an illusion of security and irresponsibility. They rendered themselves subordinate and struggled to remain as such.

Finally, there are the leaders themselves. They too may have internal pulls toward overly dependent authority relations. They may have internal models of authority – assumptions toward authority that dictate how individuals assess and act within authority relationships (Kahn & Kram 1994) – that stress dependence in leader-subordinate relations. They may be pulled toward a personally familiar role of provider or savior. They may have their own unmet needs for caregiving, which get transposed into overly dependent relations with subordinates: unable or unwilling to create relationships in which they receive care, they create relationships in which others must attend carefully to them, as subordinates do to superiors. They thus receive attention, and a vicarious if unsatisfying experience of caregiving.

Such pulls toward overly dependent relationships exert a certain amount of pressure upon both leaders and members. The pressure can be quite strong. People can make certain choices in the face of it. They can be swept along into relations of abject dependency, they can turn their backs on dependency and create relations where authority seemingly matters little, or they can withstand the pressure and try to create partnerships in which reasonable dependency needs are met in ways that enable members to retain personal integrity and authority. These parallel the choices that caregivers routinely face in negotiating the dependency of careseekers, who naturally regress as they take up the roles of students, patients, congregants, and clients. Like caregivers working with careseekers, leaders can create insecure or secure attachments with members. The former marks cultures of immature dependence; the latter marks cultures of mature dependence.

Immature dependence

There are two primary forms of immature dependence in caregiving organizations. Both take their power from the sustained memory of the parent-child relationship that underlies people's experiences of and wishes about caregiving organizations (Kahn & Kram 1994). In the first form, members and leaders embrace that relationship by embracing the leader's authority and the members' lack thereof. Members and leaders operate from a collective model of dependence. In the second form, they rebel against that relationship and seek to banish authority altogether. Members and leaders operate from a collective model of counter-dependence. Each of these is an immature dependence, for in each the leader remains at the center, a figure to be embraced or rejected. The alternative – mature dependence – involves leaders and members working with one another in some form of partnership, from a collective model of interdependence.

Dependence

Members and leaders may sustain the often unconscious, collusive belief that all authority and responsibility lies with leaders. They may collude in believing that the role of the leader is that of the parent. Leaders must provide for all needs. They must protect their followers from danger. They must give comfort upon demand. They must provide resources. For their part, members must follow the dictates and demands of their leaders. They must be followers, in the fashion of children, who submit to the will of their parent-leaders. If all play their roles, the illusion holds, all will survive. It is within those role relations that people "find themselves," and outside those relations in which they feel "lost." They follow scripts attached to hierarchical roles that offer characters to portray (i.e., stereotypical characters of "boss" and "employee"), lines to say, and plays to enact (Kahn & Kram 1994). This model echoes the anxious resistant pattern of attachment (Bowlby 1980), in which infants uncertain about the availability of parents or primary caregivers tend to cling to those figures. These infants have anxiety about exploring their world and wish to remain connected to authority figures.

This is, of course, a sub-text. Members and leaders do not make explicit their parent-child demands and expectations. They go about their work together, speaking the text of tasks and projects and outcomes. But the sub-text makes itself known in various ways. It is most visible when members look to their leaders to do for them what they as normally functioning adults ought to do themselves. They behave as if they cannot think and act for themselves. A group of nurses makes a desultory attempt to sort out the schedule for a holiday shift and then leave it for a nurse manager already preoccupied with hiring and training responsibilities. Middle managers at a large hospital protest that they do not know enough about their department budgets to develop cost-cutting measures. Teachers of a high school interdisciplinary honors course are unable to decide on a curriculum and leave it to the vice-principal to develop solutions. Social workers at a state agency decide they cannot figure out how to implement a new policy and demand that their executive director rewrite the policy for them. In such cases, organization members "de-skill" themselves. They look to their leaders – expectantly, beseechingly, or angrily – to act upon their behalf, and the leaders comply.

The sub-text is also visible when leaders act as if their followers have little to offer. The medical director of a healthcare facility issues pronouncements about policy changes, new clinical practices, and staffing schedules without bothering to ask nurses and physicians for information and suggestions. A school principal changes the physical education curriculum by fiat. The executive director of a nursing home creates a new program for residents without involving the nursing and rehabilitation staff in assessing its desirability or feasibility. A hospital CEO asks for input from his staff on changing programs to fit a new patient population and changing health regulations, but acts before the suggestions are even made. In such cases organization leaders behave as if they must think and act on behalf of others; it is as if they alone are responsible, capable, and competent. They own the authority that would otherwise be dispersed throughout their units or organizations. They are the all-knowing parental figures. They may be benign, ruling with wisdom and compassion, or they may be excessively authoritarian, imposing their will indiscriminately. Both are regimes in which leaders rule and members are ruled.

The immaturity of this culture stems from its inability to enable members and leaders alike to evolve, to grow past the limitations they set upon themselves and others. Leaders are unable to develop their followers' capacities to think and act for themselves. They do their work for them. They become over-involved, to the extent that they, rather than their followers, exist at the center of their follower's work lives. The leader's authority intrudes upon and subsumes that of the follower. The next generation of leaders cannot be developed; members learn only to be followers. They are de-skilled by themselves and their leaders alike. Their critical faculties remain underdeveloped. They are believers, defined by Memmi (1974: 39) as "[people] who, having a need to believe, will believe regardless of the argument against it." Leaders are also unable to learn and grow, shut off as they are from new information, perspectives, and challenges to their habits of thought and action. They too are believers: they believe in the inability of their followers to be competent. The caregiving organization, like the family where parents are unable to cede control and children are unable to seek and accept their own personal authority, becomes stifling to leaders and members alike.

The continued existence of this culture relates to its use as a social defense. Like Bion's (1961) basic assumption dependency groups, it is sustained by the wish to believe that omnipotent leaders will save members from uncertainty, anxiety and threats to existence. Members and leaders unconsciously collude to act as if those leaders are powerful enough to meet all their needs for survival. Members huddle together under the metaphoric shelter of their leaders. In so doing, they re-create what Memmi (1974) terms the "fundamental duet" of the parent-child relationship. Fearing separation from all-powerful figures, they do what they can to ensure that they will not be left alone. They act helpless. They provoke guilt. They create crises. They refuse to act as mature adults capable of thinking and acting responsibly. They thrust themselves and their needs upon their leaders and demand satisfaction.

The needs of such believers cannot, of course, be fully met by any leader. The task is impossible. In caregiving organizations in particular, there will always be anxiety. There will always be situations in which leaders are not sure what to do. They must routinely choose among imperfect options that have negative as well as positive implications. They will make mistakes. And they will follow various organizational and personal agendas that do not always have at their most central point the meeting of their followers' needs for reassurance and security. "There is always a margin between what is asked and what is offered," writes Memmi (1974: 48), "between the hopes, which are unlimited, and the response, which is necessarily relative." This margin provides evidence of leaders' fallibility. Among their followers, of course, there will be those who will ignore this evidence, unwilling to admit to conscious awareness the illusions they have sustained. Others, however, will attend quite intently to real or imagined evidence of betrayal. Their disappointment and frustration – their sense of betrayal – becomes woven into the tapestry of emotions that mark dependency cultures. "In that always gaping trench," continues Memmi (1974: 48), "desires proliferate, crazed by false expectations and wild figments of the imagination. That trench is also where the dependent's resentment and, often, the provider's guilt begin to develop."

A regime's ability to change requires both members and leaders to change how they relate to one another. Members need to assume their own adult functioning and not act as if they are unable to think, plan, reflect, and do for themselves. They must give up their illusory beliefs in the power of their leaders to protect them from all harm, from anxiety, indeed, from all manner of difficult emotions and experiences. There is no such protection; there is only resilience, which is generated by more mature functioning. Unless members give up their illusory beliefs about leaders, they will consent to remain always longing, always resentful, always enslaved. Even if their current authoritarian leaders were to be deposed, they would, in time, cast another into the same leader role and themselves into the same relationship of abject dependence. "This is central to the dependency culture," writes Miller (1993: 312). "There has to be the parental figure to receive the projections of love/ hate, responsibility, and blame." It is only when members are willing to take responsibility for what occurs that they will allow a different type of leader. Similarly, it is only when leaders are willing to share responsibility that they will allow a different type of member to emerge.

Counter-dependence

Members and leaders may also distance themselves from dependency needs altogether. They embrace their wish that members are completely autonomous and self-reliant and have no emotional needs for leaders to meet. The role of the leader is that of the strategist, not the parent. The role of the member is that of the independent contractor, not the child. On the surface, their relationships are marked less by longing than by a distance between adults who expect, and receive, little from one another. Beneath the surface, however, the leader's authority is minimized, undermined and devalued by members whose needs for support remain unexpressed and unmet. This model echoes the anxious avoidant pattern of attachment (Bowlby 1980), in which infants without confidence in, and expecting rejection from, parents or primary caregivers distance themselves from those figures. These infants have become emotionally self-sufficient and suppress their needs for help from authority figures. Authority figures collude by remaining unavailable.

This form of immature dependence makes itself known in several ways in caregiving organizations. Members deny their needs for assistance or support. Nurses, social workers, and childcare workers work their shifts, go home, and try to forget or deny how much they would have liked supervisors and managers to help them feel better about upsetting situations. Middle managers running hospital units act as if they have no need for senior executives to help them develop strategies, deal with unfamiliar situations, or console them about recent failures. People thus withhold their own needs. They do so for any number of reasons. They may try and protect leaders from having to contend with difficult emotions and anxieties, or leaders may have previously proven themselves unavailable, unwilling, or unable to deal with others' needs, leaving members unwilling to risk disappointment and rejection. When leaders do not draw members out and take seriously their needs for support, they collude with members' beliefs in their leaders' inability or unwillingness to provide such support.

When members deny their needs they may turn their anger inwards, ultimately harming themselves. Or they may express anger directly at their leaders, resisting them or seeking to drive them away altogether. A group of schoolteachers write letters to the school superintendent protesting the lack of supervision by their principal. Agency social workers speak disrespectfully to their executive director, furious at his inability to conduct useful performance reviews, hire a competent supervisor, or treat their requests for assistance seriously. In such cases, people express rather than deny their anger. They do so directly, in confrontations, or more passively, circumventing leaders' authority without challenging it directly. They assume roles – as resisters, gossips, rebels, blockers – through which they express resentment toward authority. For some, however, the depth of their anger is related to the depth of their disappointed hopes and longings; they wished to believe in the hope and illusion of the leader's omnipotence, and unable to sustain that illusion, now turn against their leaders. For others, their anger is related to the shame and fear evoked in them by dependency (Hirschhorn 1997), which gets compounded when their needs are ignored or dismissed.

Members and leaders may also create overly personal relationships and minimize role and status differences to avoid expressing or meeting reasonable dependency needs. A group of social workers befriend their new supervisor, going out drinking and dancing after work. A nurse dates her supervisor. A teacher has regular social engagements with her vice-principal, their families often getting together on weekends. A hospital CEO regularly goes golfing with a department head. On the surface these personal relationships simply enable people to get to know and trust one another. However, when their formal roles drop away at work and are subsumed by their personal relationships, something else entirely lies beneath the surface. Leader and member are then colluding to obliterate their authority relationship and in doing so they unconsciously move away from what makes them uncomfortable, namely, the expressing and meeting of real dependency needs at work. This strategy may also be rooted in members' distrust, anger, and disappointment in their leaders' ability to meet those needs. It is also rooted in the leaders' own wishes to step away from having to meet those needs.

Leaders and members each sustain counter-dependent cultures. Leaders distance themselves from members. They create overly bureaucratic relations. They respond badly to members' requests for emotional support. They intimidate, brush off, and ignore members. Or they seduce members emotionally, subsuming their needs in favor of the leader's needs. In such ways, leaders abandon members. For their part, members protect leaders, suppressing rather than expressing reasonable dependency needs. They pretend that their leaders are simply their friends. Or they express anger, passively or directly, toward their leaders in ways designed to drive their leaders away. Such dynamics sustain cultures in which members' needs remain unmet.

Counter-dependent cultures are marked by a series of interrelated perceptions. Members perceive leaders as distant, out of touch, uncaring. Or they perceive them as nice but ineffectual. These perceptions drive self-fulfilling prophecies. Members suppress or withhold their needs for support and then dismiss or rail against their leaders for not meeting those needs. For their part, leaders perceive members as self-sufficient and therefore do not regularly attempt to provide support. They perceive members as enraged and petulant, driving away attempts at support. Or they perceive them as colleagues and friends. These perceptions also become the basis for self-fulfilling prophecies. Leaders remove themselves from the equation, acting as if members either do not need or cannot accept their help. This simply confirms members' perceptions and the two remain locked within a cycle of mutually self-fulfilling prophecies.

This culture also owes its continued existence to its use as a social defense. It is sustained by people's wish to believe that by ignoring dependency needs they will disappear. People ignore them by mobilizing rebellion against authority, in direct confrontation or passive withdrawal. These are, in Bion's (1961) terms, responses to anger at authority: active, rebellion is the "fight" response, passive withdrawal the "flight" response. In the former, organization members struggle to topple the authority structure and their places within it; in the latter they deny its existence altogether. Caught up in such struggles, members and leaders unconsciously seek to avoid anxiety associated with their primary tasks. Indeed, they wish to believe that if dependency needs are not expressed, anxiety cannot exist. The reality, of course, is that individuals with real dependency needs are not attended to; they are left as casualties of the counter-dependent culture.

Mature dependence

Each of the two forms of immature dependency cultures represents a choice that leaders and members implicitly make about how to negotiate dependency needs. When they choose to act as if leaders are parents and members are children, they are negotiating terms of surrender to authority. When they choose to act as if members are completely autonomous and self-reliant and leaders are fragile, untrustworthy or withholding, they are negotiating terms of escape from authority. Each of these enables people to avoid the difficult work of creating relationships in which leaders and members are both related to and autonomous from one another. In the overly dependent culture they are too related: leaders intrude upon members who have little autonomy, who invite intrusion through their own eager acceptance of others' authority. In the counter-dependent culture they are too autonomous: leaders abandon members who receive little support, who invite abandonment by suppressing their needs and resisting or ignoring others' authority.

There is another choice, however. Caregiving organizations or their units may create cultures of *mature dependence*. This is marked by a collective healthy respect for both autonomy and relatedness. Members are believed to have the capacity to think and act for themselves. Leaders are believed to have the capacity to provide useful support in appropriate ways and at appropriate times. These shared beliefs enable members and leaders to create useful partnerships, in which, like healthy marriages, they at times operate separately, each attending to particular tasks, and at other times join for support, planning and action. Underlying these beliefs is a fundamental assumption woven into the culture of a caregiving system: that people may temporarily regress in the face of anxiety and troubling emotions while still retaining basic adult capacities for thought and action.

This assumption lies at the heart of the mature dependency culture in caregiving organizations. Leaders and members alike are aware of the need for those who work most closely with careseekers to temporarily regress. Nurses working a cancer ward inevitably get filled with sadness, guilt, anger, and hope. They need to feel those emotions. They need respite from their patients. They need various outlets for releasing emotions – talking, joking, playing, mourning, celebrating. They need their unit director to create or support such outlets and to create places – in her office, in staff meetings, in formal and informal gatherings – in which they can safely do what they need to do to release emotions and regain composure and compassion. Mostly, they need their director to hold onto the belief in their capacities to return to their work as mature, functioning adults, even as they safely give in to the depths of their emotions somewhere off-stage. Gathering themselves, they exit the wings, re-enter the stage, and take up their work. Their dependency needs appropriately met, they can see to those of their patients.

Similar descriptions can be written for teachers in relation to their students filling them with anxiety about the future, anger at and longing for authority, and confusion about personal and sexual identities. They may be written for clergy filled with others' anxieties and despair about the nature and meaning of death and its relation to life. They may be written for childcare workers filled with anger, sadness and hopelessness in relation to parents and families who inflict emotional or physical damage upon children. In mature dependent relations the leader tends to staff filled with complicated emotions. Proactively or reactively, the leader enables members to safely release anxieties and emotions. Yet this remains only one part of leaders' tasks, one strand of their relationship with members. That relationship does not become so dominated by members' longings for help that they become blind to the other aspects of their leaders' roles, or for that matter, so dominated by leaders' longings to help or avoid that they become blind to members' adult capacities or their reasonable needs for support.

Such longings never really disappear. Caregiving organization members will always be torn between longing for their leaders to make their anxiety go away and wishing to believe they themselves are completely self-sufficient. Caregiving organization leaders will always be torn between trying to save members from pain and wanting to turn away from it entirely. These are human impulses. How those impulses are worked with determines whether people create mature or immature dependency relations. People giving into their longings mark the latter. Leaders get seduced by their own wishes to rescue members, who indulge their own fantasies of saviors keeping them safe or suffering on their behalf. Or leaders give in to their impulses to flee, believing that they can run from anxiety and pain completely, while members believe their own illusions of self-sufficiency. People may be swept away by their longings for the impossible.

In mature dependency relations, something quite different occurs. People retain their awareness of the limits of what others can do in the face of anxiety, pain, and suffering. They realize that leaders are not parents who can simply pick them up like small children and with a kiss or a bandage make their hurts disappear. They realize that anxiety, uncertainty, and troubling emotions are inevitable aspects of their work and cannot be made to disappear. They realize, finally, that it is only when people join together to face the reality of their experiences that the troubling aspects of their work can be worked *with* and (to the extent possible) mitigated and relieved.

The mature leader's stance

These realizations begin, often enough, with leaders themselves. When they adopt a certain stance toward their tasks, members and themselves, they can help move people and units toward mature dependence. The stance requires maturity on their part: the knowledge, ability, and willingness to face squarely and knowingly difficult responsibilities and choices and discharge them according to what ought to be done for the health of the system and its careseekers.

Mature dependence is thus created and maintained in part by a leader's devotion to a primary task and the conviction that it can only be achieved when adults work together across roles and responsibilities. The leader's stance is thus anchored in the singular pursuit of the primary task. As Miller (1993: 313) notes:

> The leadership required of management is to define the task and to equip groups and individuals with the requisite resources so that they can manage themselves to perform it. If in that way the task itself becomes the leader, hallowed concepts such as subordination, obedience, and personal loyalty become outmoded and are replaced by negotiation between adults responsible for managing the boundaries of their respective systems and sub-systems.

Miller describes the *task* as the leader, followed by organization members inhabiting various roles. Mature leaders believe exactly that. They believe that adults capable of taking and defending positions based on what they believe to be in the best interests of patients, students, clients, or congregants must inhabit the organization. System members must devote themselves not to their leaders but to attending to careseekers' needs.

This will occur to the extent leaders are able to assume different aspects of the leadership role. There will be times, of course, when they need to take action. A school headmaster fires a teacher who committed an ethical impropriety. A residential treatment center director renegotiates a reimbursement schedule with state agencies. A hospital unit director adds staff for weekend shifts. Such leadership helps to protect boundaries, sets strategy, or adds resources. At other times, leaders need to facilitate. They convene staff members, pose problems and help them develop and implement solutions. A headteacher calls together others in the English literature department and says parents are complaining that their children are not getting enough writing assignments to prepare for college admissions. She facilitates a problem-solving discussion resulting in a solution different to the one she herself would have imagined. The chief of surgery of a local hospital calls together the staff and says that a certain medical procedure is taking more time than seems necessary and he's not sure why. He facilitates a conversation among the nurses and surgeons, who come up with a plan to try a different anesthesia set-up. The power of the leader's role here is directly related to their willingness to hold tightly to the aim of developing solutions to pressing problems but not to a preferred solution. Members are thus pointed toward a goal but they must engage their own critical faculties, together, to reach that goal.

Leaders need to facilitate not only problem-solving but also the expression and productive channeling of anxiety. They must supervise, in the clinical sense of the term. As described in Chapter 3, resilient caregiving systems are marked by flows of supervision. Leaders are the linchpins of those systems. They must be able to sit with their staff, singly or in groups, and enable them to speak of their experiences. The residential director at a treatment center debriefs the staff at a residential house whose clients have just staged a terrible fight. The minister of a church sits with a staff member whose new program to combat poverty is failing. The executive director of a homeless shelter listens to two new staff discuss their experiences of being isolated by veteran staff members. These leaders provide holding environments. They enable others to let loose their emotions – the residential staff's guilt and anger, the church staff member's confusion and sadness, the homeless staff members' isolation and anger. They help members develop possible solutions without taking on members' problems as their own to solve. They quite deliberately try to develop members' capacities to examine their own experiences and make sense of them, and using those insights, develop effective courses of action.

These leaders are in effect pulling for others to bring to the surface their own mature capacities for thought and action. They understand that this requires a temporary regression. Members must first express how guilty or sad or furious they are, their confusion and uncertainty about what has occurred and what they ought to do about it. This is a step away from the calmly rational discourse that marks most work-related conversations. Once members have taken this step, leaders can help them diagnose situations and develop strategies. They pose questions. They offer insight and feedback. They suggest experiments. They engage members as partners and collaborators, as fellow detectives in the pursuit of knowledge about troubling situations and their resolutions. Implicit in this process is leaders modeling for others expressing rather than acting out anxiety: they are *modeling resilience*.

This requires leaders themselves to exhibit certain qualities. They must contain rather than act out their own anxiety. When they feel anxious they do not try and get members to feel it on their behalf, directly (by inappropriately telling others of their fears) or indirectly (by treating others in ways that make them anxious). At the same time, mature leaders are open and accessible, and within limits, vulnerable in their dealings with system members. A clinical supervisor dries her tears as her staff tell her of a physically abused child. The chief of emergency medicine is upset when a staff member reports that a patient's family member removed him before tests were complete. A school headmaster chuckles during a staff meeting at which a teacher tells an anecdote about a favored student. At such moments leaders are interacting as fellow human beings. They show themselves to be vulnerable to natural human emotion, affected by staff and careseekers alike. They do this within boundaries, however, so as not to force others to have to watch out for or take care of them and neglect their own needs and work.

Leaders must also remain curious. When people are genuinely curious, they allow themselves and others to explore multiple explanations for events. They do not lock others into particular, projected identities that constrain their abilities to learn and grow (Shapiro & Carr 1991). When leaders are curious, members feel *worked with* rather than *judged*. They feel safer in discussing what they are thinking and feeling, how they are approaching situations, what steps they are planning to take – exactly what leaders need to know in order to coach others toward more effective ways to think and act.

When leaders are themselves openly self-reflective, examining their own thoughts and feelings, curious as to what they might reveal, they offer models that enlarge further the possibilities for coaching. A supervisor in a residential treatment center for adolescents reflects during a staff meeting her recent insight about how a bout of anger at the agency's executive director had little to do with the director and much to do with how angry she was at parents who had done so much damage. This enabled other staff to acknowledge that they too were often upset with the executive director and the entire administrative team and did not know what to do with that anger. The supervisor shared her own strategies, some of which involved finding trusted peers and administrators to confide in and from whom to receive feedback. She helped staff develop their own strategies. Her self-reflections, made public, provided the impetus for a coaching session that offered the opportunity for others to develop insight and changed behaviors. Key to this process is the leader's own vulnerability. When leaders can surface or be confronted with their own limitations, they enable others to have, in Balint's memorable phrase, "the courage of [their] own stupidity"(1968).

The mature leader's stance is, finally, anchored in the belief that it is the task, not themselves, that ought to be at the center of awareness. This requires humility. Members will look to leaders instinctively, based on the pulls toward dependence that mark caregiving organizations. Mature leaders are appropriately wary of members' longings to be taken care of. They do not take those longings personally, as if they really are the saviors that members seek. They recognize the value of the dependency needs that others justly have and seek to meet them appropriately, but they remain a respectful distance from needy gravitational pull, lest they become trapped in becoming the leader who intrudes upon or abandons others. They resist becoming indispensable. They resist keeping themselves central, to be longed for or fended off by members. They focus on enabling others to develop their own capacities for rational, mature thought and action. They do this in part out of self-preservation, to fend off others' incessant longings, disappointment, and senses of deprivation. But they also do it because they understand that it is the path toward people living reasonably well with anxiety. Resilience is created through the bringing together of as many functioning adults as possible to bear and work through anxiety, uncertainty, and painful affect.

Leaders thus need to let others occupy the center of their own work lives while they themselves recede into a more bounded, less intrusive, supportive role. This can be a difficult transformation. Some leaders wish to believe in their own abilities to save others, for reasons related to their own personal needs and histories. Others do not wish to let go of the power accorded them. They exist at the apex of a system's hierarchy and enjoy the privileges therein, and for this they pay a heavy price. They are the object of constant longing and constant hostility. Members yearn for an endless supply of resources; they yearn for the leader's touch, presence, love; they are furious when it is not forthcoming; and they resort to continued manipulations to coax, seduce, or force the leader into the parental role or out of the system entirely. Mature leaders refuse to play this game. They refuse to collude with members' need – and their own, for that matter – to believe in their own omnipotence.

Playing for keeps

The struggle to resolve the knotty question of dependency is crucial to the creation of an effective caregiving organization. The outcomes of that struggle affect not only the organization but also its careseekers. The parallel processes that mark these systems make it likely that relations at one level of the organization will mirror or create models for relations at other levels. When leaders and members are locked into immature dependency relations they *invariably* re-create those relations with careseekers. When they create mature dependency relations they *often* re-create those relations with careseekers. Relations between leaders and members may thus be a significant intervention, a vehicle by which careseekers are helped to engage their own mature functioning, to the extent that they are truly capable in the service of their own healing, growing, and learning. They may also simply be re-enactments of careseekers' own immature dependent relations, their own abject longings for, resentful denials of, or withdrawals from, help. Uninterrupted, these may hold sway in relations throughout the caregiving organization.

Leaders thus play a large role in determining whether their relations with members facilitate or undermine the mature dependence of careseekers. Leaders can provide members with their own opportunities to grow and develop at work. They give them responsibility and hold them accountable while providing them with the appropriate training, tools, resources, and support to enable them to succeed. They offer them autonomy. All of this calls forth the mature, adult functioning of staff members. This has direct bearing on calling forth the mature functioning of careseekers, to the extent that is possible, in that caregivers offer models, intentionally and not, of mature or immature functioning. In caregiving organizations, careseekers attend closely to how staff members take up their roles – the degrees of autonomy, self-reliance, and ability to seek and receive help – as clues to how they themselves ought to take up their own tasks of learning, growing, and healing (Lyth 1988).

Leaders therefore accomplish several goals by enabling members to experience both autonomy and support. First, of course, they gain partners in raising and solving problems. Second, staff members experience what it means to be in relations of mature dependence; they know what it feels like to be both responsible for oneself and able to ask for and receive support from others when anxious or overwhelmed. They are then more likely to be able to facilitate that experience in others for whom they themselves are responsible. Third, they are able to tolerate without envy others' growth and development. Some caregivers, as noted earlier, join their organizations because of their own unmet needs for nurturing and support. They may be thus susceptible to envying those whose needs are well met. When their own maturity is valued, however, and they themselves have the opportunity to grow, they are more likely to value and encourage others' growth.

Effective leaders thus intellectually or intuitively grasp the intimate relation between how they negotiate their members' twin needs for autonomy and support and how those members negotiate careseekers' dependency needs. They understand that their own relations with organization members offer a singular tool by which to shape careseekers' experiences. They constantly recalibrate their distance from staff members, finding and losing and finding again the appropriate balances between remaining too close (intruding upon) and staying too far away from (abandoning) members. They understand that staff members who feel overly controlled will unconsciously seek to shift those experiences onto careseekers; and that staff members who feel abandoned and isolated will unconsciously seek to induce those feelings within careseekers. They understand, finally, the need to press for a system of caregiving by which their respect for both the maturity and regression of staff members is reproduced for careseekers.

Chapter 13

Leadership and change

Caregiving organizations are subject to pressures to change what and how they provide for careseekers. Changing client populations, regulations and policies, and markets force leaders to develop and implement new strategies. Serious errors, intergroup conflicts, leadership successions, and other disruptions of organizational life press people to change how they work. Organizations must thus adapt to new realities in their social, political, economic, or cultural contexts or within their own interiors. If these new realities are not worked with in some useful way – confronted, figured out, integrated, managed – organizations and their members will struggle. Old strategies for attracting and retaining careseekers will no longer be effective. Difficult issues within and between units will grow more complicated and fracture organizations. Careseekers' needs will be met less effectively.

Such struggles and their ill effects are signs that change is necessary. They signal some disturbance in how members work with one another or serve careseekers, or in how they interpret and react to their contexts. Such signals may not be attended to. People may construct narratives to explain away disturbing patterns. They may tell themselves stories that help them dismiss situations or trends they should examine more carefully. Such stories may remain current for quite some time. They may become woven into organizational cultures, attaining the status of accepted facts. Yet signals may get louder, more insistent. Near misses in a medical setting – medication errors caught by nurses, misidentified patients saved by medical residents – occur more frequently or become fully-fledged errors. Restraints in a residential setting occur more often or forcefully, until a client is seriously injured. Isolated discipline problems in a classroom lead to pitched battles between a teacher and her class. In each case, people are sending signals of some underlying disturbance to which organization leaders and members must attend. Often enough, they do not do so until they have no choice, and until solutions become drastic and costly.

A tenet of *transformational change* – that is, change that is not simply cosmetic or temporary – is that people rarely seek it out unless there is pain or the threat thereof. Organizations experience pain when they are losing money, market share, programs, or clients. Groups and teams experience pain when their work is unacceptable. Individuals experience pain when their work experiences are unsatisfactory or emotionally difficult, or when they are in danger of losing what is important to them. With enough actual or potential pain, people may decide to look beneath the surface of the stories they routinely tell themselves and begin to examine the social defenses they have constructed. Such defenses, as described throughout this book, distort people's views and experiences of their work (Jacques 1974; Lyth 1988; Obholzer 1994). They prevent them from seeing and responding clearly to their environments, one another, and careseekers. Pain or its possibility, however, may press people to look at rather than through the lenses of their defenses. It may press them to deconstruct those defenses.

Then again, they may not. While pain generates the need for change it also mobilizes familiar defenses. People may cling to their accepted ways of thinking and acting in the hope that those habits may, like a talisman, protect them from harm. They may do this at great cost to themselves and those they attempt to help. As Lyth (1988: 62) wrote about the nursing ward in her classic study, "In order to avoid anxiety, the service tries to avoid change wherever possible – almost, one might say, at all costs – and tends to cling to the familiar even when the familiar has obviously ceased to be appropriate or relevant. Changes tend to be initiated only at the point of crisis." When pain turns into full-blown crises, people face a stark choice: they can hold onto their habits of thought and action, and risk faring badly amidst their crises, or they can move toward change and more anxiety without the distorting protection of familiar social defenses. This is not an easy choice. Its resolution often determines the outcomes of organizational change efforts.

The underlying assumption here is that meaningful, lasting change – that which transforms rather than simply restates how organizations and their members think about and perform their work – cannot occur without some dismantling of social defenses (Lyth 1988; Miller 1993; Rice 1963). Organizational change occurs at two levels: substantive (changes in products, services, clients, programs, or structures) and relational (changes in relationships within and across organizational boundaries). With only substantive changes, organizations do different things but may not do things differently. Without relational changes, the familiar ways in which people limit themselves and one another at work remain even if they present differently. Transformational change occurs when substantive changes are accompanied by supporting relational changes. Relational changes, ideally, involve people creating increasingly effective ways of using one another to cope with anxiety at work. Without such shifts, people cannot fully and effectively solve problems, develop strategy, and support one another during and after change processes.

This chapter focuses on the process of changing caregiving organizations. One premise, as elsewhere in this book, is that work relationships in these organizations must have the capacity for resilience. Transformational change must therefore occur in ways that enable caregiving organization members to build upon, strengthen, or repair relations within and across various groups, the better to withstand the inevitable stress of working with careseekers. This echoes the premise of family systems theory, which focuses on transforming destructive patterns of interaction into constructive patterns that leave family members supporting one another in stressful situations and transitions (Byng-Hall 1998). Similarly, without the creation of such capacities for resilience, organizational change efforts are likely to remain superficial, be incremental rather than transformative, or fail altogether as members retreat behind distorting social defenses. Simultaneous movements toward change and toward self-protection will compete for people's hearts and minds, with self-protection winning more often than not.

This chapter also addresses the role of leaders in the change process. Leaders can help others interrupt dysfunctional, self-limiting patterns of behavior. They can make transparent and discussable less functional aspects of group and organizational life. They can model and lead the examination of social defenses, and they can attend to the emotional life of their organizations. Effective leaders understand that beneath the layer of observable organizational behavior run streams of emotions that shape how people think, feel, and act. They have some understanding of how those emotional undercurrents are shaped by the needs and emotions of careseekers. They sense the power of these emotional undercurrents, how they move people toward and away from one another in useful and less useful ways and ideally act on the basis of such understandings. They attempt to develop their members' capacities to reflect upon, learn from, and interrupt the breakdown of underlying systems of caregiving.

Organizational maturation

Transformational change in caregiving organizations, in addition to reshaping what and how careseekers' needs are met, ideally creates or reinforces organizational cultures, processes, and structures that press members toward healthy, functional responses to distress. Such organizations are *mature*. The meaning of this term is described in some detail here, for the maturity of a social system is intimately related to its capacity for resilience. Transformational change in social systems both depends upon and enables such maturation.

George Valliant (1993: 115), a psychologist specializing in adult development, offers a useful description of maturity. He writes:

> Maturity is many things. Maturity includes having appropriate expectations and goals for oneself and finding a major source of fulfillment in productive work. Maturity includes the capacity to love and to hope. It includes the ability to discharge hostility without harming others or

oneself, and the capacity to suspend one's adult identity and engage in childlike play. Finally, maturity includes the capacity to adapt to change, to endure frustrations and loss, and to maintain an altruistic concern for human beings outside one's own group and beyond one's own time and place.

This description may be adapted to describe the maturity of social systems as well, in this case, of caregiving organizations and their units. Organizational cultures may enable members, as a matter of course, to find fulfillment in productive work, to experience hope and hostility without harm, to play, to adapt, to experience loss, and to forge altruistic connections with others. Such cultures are mature. They are resilient, enabling their members to work with and through distressing situations and experiences.

The transformational change of caregiving organizations involves creating such mature systems. Paradoxically, such change also depends in part on such maturity already existing. To withstand the tremors and quakes of change – the anxiety inherent in the loss of habits of thought and action – organization members need some capacity for hope, for the discharge of hostility, for play; they need to endure frustration and loss while adapting to new ideas, behaviors, and relationships. They need maturity. Every organization member need not have reached the highest levels of adult development, rather, their units or organizations must have cultures that press them, through norms and expectations, toward such behaviors. The cultures guide and sustain them as they engage in the work of changing what and how they provide for careseekers. Mature cultures provide meaning and momentum for the maturation of their members.

Mature social systems – relationships, families, groups, and organizations – are marked by two subtle but crucial characteristics that are routinely at play but assert themselves dramatically during times of transition and change. The first is the dispersion of pain and hope, such that all members have access to both. The second is the use of mature defenses by people to cope with painful situations. These characteristics are described below, as they apply to caregiving organizations.

Dispersion of pain and hope

Pain suffuses caregiving organizations; it is brought in from careseekers, triggered within organization members, or imported from the environment. Such pain, when it becomes too costly, spurs change efforts, as people attempt to move toward some less painful circumstances. In immature systems, change processes are relatively superficial and consigned to relatively small areas. Pain spreads neither far nor deeply. Individuals, sub-groups or units bear a disproportionate amount of the pain, and change efforts focus on them specifically rather than on the larger systems in which they are embedded (see Frost 2003). At Project Home (Chapter 5), the social workers bore the brunt of careseekers' pain, cut off as they were from the other parts of the agency. At Greenvale Residential Treatment Center (Chapter 7), the department heads contained pain on behalf of subordinates and superiors alike. At Sudbury Hospital (Chapter 8), the ER unit was left alone with the pain of its client population, as other hospital units and senior administrators withdrew. At Maple Hospital (Chapter 10), the nurse manager of the SU was left to contain the pain from an earlier unit trauma. In each case, specific individuals or groups were casualties, sacrificed by their organizations in lieu of deeper systemic changes.

Family systems theorists refer to such casualties as "identified patients" that families unconsciously select to contain and present problems that exist unacknowledged in the family unit itself. As Friedman (1985: 19) writes, "The concept of the identified patient is that the family member with the obvious symptom is to be seen not as the 'sick one' but as the one in whom the family stress or pathology has surfaced." The family seeks to isolate the seemingly problematic member from the overall relationship system of the family, as if the two are unrelated. This "enables the rest of the family to 'purify' itself by locating the source of its 'disease' in the disease of the identified patient" (Friedman 1985: 20). The individual member is sacrificed, in the way that an individual limb is sacrificed by a tourniquet that cuts off its blood flow while temporarily preserving the rest of the body. The system itself resists real change. As Friedman notes (p. 20), "When one part of the organism is treated in isolation from its interconnections with another, as though the problem were solely its own, fundamental change is not likely. The symptom is apt to recycle, in the same or different form, in the same or different member." The system continues to cycle through its members, scapegoating and sacrificing them in the futile hope of making the pain go away.

In mature systems, however, pain is dispersed such that no member or group holds more than their fair share. Individuals or groups that emerge as problematic are examined for what they signal about the functioning of systems themselves. At Project Home (Chapter 5), the social workers would have been worked with until they and the administrators understood the abandonment and isolation they "re-presented" from their clients' experiences. At Greenvale Residential Treatment Center (Chapter 7), the department heads would have joined with the administrative team to learn about how their struggles with one another were rooted in the lack of a shared model of a multidisciplinary therapeutic milieu. At Sudbury Hospital (Chapter 8), the ER leaders, with facilitation from senior hospital administrators, would have worked with their peers in other units to create a more effective system for admitting patients. At Maple Hospital (Chapter 10), senior administrators would have helped the SU nurse manager understand what she was acting out on behalf of the unit, and then convened members to examine how their current relationships were in reaction to previous traumatic events. In each case the system rather than its seemingly problematic members becomes the focus of change efforts.

Such a process depends on the dispersion of pain. Members who are not seemingly affected by others' difficulties make themselves affected: they come close to rather than distance themselves from others, looking for ways in which they contributed to those others' difficulties. This requires the liberal use of empathy, with members actively seeking to see themselves in others; this is the opposite of projective identification, which involves denying one's empathic connections with others. The lack of projective identification marks such relationships as mature (Fairbairn 1952); in immature relationships, a person "not only fails to acknowledge the pain of others but also leaves his or her own pain within other people to fester and to be regarded as their own" (Vaillant 1993: 272). In mature relationships, people strike the stance of what Hinshelwood (2001: 88) terms "involved witnessing," an "experience [of] an 'as if I were them' state whilst holding in reserve a knowledge that one is not in fact them."

In mature systems, people thus witness one another closely enough to share their pain without being disabled by it. They take in others' pain and offer something in return as well: hope. In mature systems, hope is dispersed as well as pain; in immature systems some people bear disproportionate amounts of hope while others bear disproportionate pain (cf. Frost 2003). When hope is spread throughout a system it offers an antidote to potentially debilitating pain; it enables members to engage a change process, to bear the pain with some sense that it can end well. Transformational change thus occurs when pain intrudes within the larger system and is made manageable by its dispersion throughout individuals and groups, none of which get so loaded up that they cannot function usefully. The dispersion of pain makes it tolerable for all system members, not just some at the expense of others. This process creates system-level resilience. As Vaillant (1993: 314) writes, "Hope and faith are very simple words, but they encompass an essential facet of resilience. It is no accident that hope has long been seen, as in the myth of Pandora, as the psychic balm on which resilience depends. And hope and faith are inextricably bound to social supports." The myth of Pandora lingers within caregiving organizations, whose members work to provide hope for careseekers seeking comfort in their struggles to learn, grow, or heal.

Vaillant refers to social supports as the basis of hope. Social support – healthy connections among unit and organization members – enables pain to be dispersed so people can bear affect together. Members join with others and struggle together to make sense of their experiences and develop ways to work effectively. They laugh together; they cry together; they swear together. They do not distort reality by locating pain in some members and hope in others. Rather, they all maintain some balance of pain and hope that enables each to experience reality fully – their victories and their losses, their sadness and joy – while striving together to create a better reality for themselves and others. This balance lies at the heart of a resilient system. Members work with others' distress and pain, or are thrust into some crisis, and they become misshapen, thinking and acting and feeling in ways they would ordinarily not. But together they right themselves. "Resilience," writes Vaillant (1993: 284), "conveys both the capacity to be bent back without breaking and the capacity, once bent, to spring back." In mature systems, the dispersion of both pain and hope enables members to "spring back."

The use of mature defenses

The dispersion of pain and hope does not make pain disappear. This is not possible. What is possible is to make it more bearable. As Miller (1993: 230) notes:

> The stress and pain of caring for the crippled, the old, the mad or the dying cannot be made to go away; but if they are articulated, then at least the burden can be distributed more widely. In this way the need for defensive structures, though not eliminated, may be reduced, and alternative systems may be found which, while catering for defensive needs, do so in a way that is less destructive.

As Miller suggests, the use of defenses are unavoidable for people involved in painful caregiving tasks. The question is how destructive they are, to people and their work with others. Mature social systems are characterized by the widespread use of less destructive, mature defenses against pain. Mature defenses enable people to not get too anxious or too depressed; they are selective self-deceptions through which people cope with otherwise unbearable experiences. This formulation represents a movement away from classic psychoanalytic theory, in that Freud saw defenses as *only* pathological: "Freud did not always appreciate that defenses were homeostatic and could help even the most psychologically healthy adult keep from being immobilized by anxiety and depression" (Vaillant 1993: 13).

Vaillant (p. 11) argues that defense mechanisms "are for the mind what the immune system is for the body." They enable people to cope with, adapt to and survive within situations that present unbearable psychological conflict or to changes too fast to accommodate. Mature defenses distort reality, but in ways that enable people to usefully integrate and manage distressing situations and experience. Vaillant describes five mature defenses. *Altruism* allows the doing for others as one would be done by, leaving the self partly gratified; *sublimation* allows the indirect or attenuated expression of instincts through action; *suppression* involves the semi-conscious decision to postpone paying attention to a conscious impulse or conflict, as when one postpones immediate gratifications; *anticipation* involves the realistic, affect-laden planning for future discomfort, thus spreading anxiety out over time; and *humor* helps keep ideas, affect, and objects in mind, enabling people to bear what is otherwise too painful. These defenses are mature to the extent that they enable people to cope, to adapt to painful or anxiety-producing circumstances. They enable people to safely bring themselves close to, rather than wall themselves off from, those circumstances. As Vaillant (1993: 104) writes, "Rather than simply anesthetize, a defense should reduce pain. Defenses should channel feelings rather than block them."

Immature defense mechanisms, on the other hand, are maladaptive and pathological. They include *projective identification*, thought processes that protect people from taking responsibility for their own feelings; *fantasy*; *hypochondriasis*; *passive aggression*, in which people turn against their own selves; *acting out*, the direct expression of unconscious wishes or impulses in order to avoid being conscious of accompanying affect; and *disassociation*, replacing painful ideas and affects with pleasant ones in order to evade depression and anxiety. These defenses distort reality in ways that push people away from taking responsibility. They are destructive to relationships:

> The use of defenses should attract people rather than repel them. The greatest distinction between the mature and immature defenses is that with the mature defenses the subject's regulatory self-deceptions are perceived by those close by as virtuous and attractive. In the case of immature defenses, such self-deceptions are seen by others as irritating, wicked, and repellent.
>
> (Vaillant 1993: 105)

The maturity of one's defenses is thus indicated by the degree to which one joins with or distances from others.

This distinction has implications for the cultures of caregiving organizations. Resilient cultures are marked by the use of defenses that enable people to join together, using the platform of empathy. "Ego development," notes Vaillant (1993: 9), "reflects our ongoing striving to allow the self-diminishing sin of projection to evolve toward the self-expanding virtue of empathy." This has its parallel at the level of social systems. Organizational cultures may press people toward diminishing themselves and others, locking all within roles (through splitting and projection) that simplify them and their relations. This characterizes many of the organizations profiled in Part 2. Other cultures may press people to support one another to expand themselves and for their relationships to contain, collectively if not individually, the full range and complexity of their experiences with careseekers and one another. These cultures, marked by the use of mature defense mechanisms, enable system-level resilience.

Engaging change

The caregiving organization leader's role involves enabling members to create increasingly mature organizations in the course of making substantive changes to programs, structures, and services. Effective leaders help members engage change at two levels simultaneously: at the observable level, the substance of the change, whether it be different programs, services, and policies; and at the underlying relational level, the dispersion of pain and hope, and the use of appropriate defenses, that mark mature (and maturing) caregiving systems. Both levels are intimately related to the success of transformational change efforts. Both are instrumental in the creation of "self-righting tendencies" for organizations and their units.

As a change agent the caregiving organization leader must attend to both levels. This involves different aspects. There are the classic steps of managing complex organizational change, such as developing visions, creating guiding coalitions, enabling participation, and the like (Kotter 1996; Lewin 1951). There is also managing the underlying emotional and relational aspects of organizational life that are inevitably stirred during significant change (Stapley 1996). The leader's role thus contains elements associated with both traditional change management (visionary, motivator, cheerleader) and the management of complex emotions and system dynamics (therapist, consultant). I now describe four key processes – *diagnosis, engagement, containment,* and *creating capacity* – by which leaders use these roles to engage transformational organizational change.

Diagnosis

At the beginning of the chapter I noted the various signs that caregiving organizations and their units emit to signal disturbances. Those signs are implicit calls for change that might ease or prevent pain. If those signals are heeded, significant change becomes possible. Leaders have a key role here. They may pick up the signals themselves – how their markets are dwindling, profits falling, morale decreasing, new ideas not forthcoming – or they may be receptive to others who interpret the signals. Either way, leaders are in the position of enabling a diagnostic process by which such signals are traced to their sources and understood as symptoms of larger issues.

The diagnostic process offers a significant opportunity for leaders to signal their willingness and ability to hold fast to primary tasks. Effective leaders focus on how those tasks get held onto or lost in members' relations with careseekers and one another. They insist on examining how group and intergroup relations, organizational structures and processes, programs and policies, the location and use of authority, and other facets of their organizations serve primary tasks. They ask others to look closely at such factors, to examine them as a physician examines a failing patient's symptoms in order to make determinations about possible underlying causes. At Project Home (Chapter 5) an effective supervisor would have examined social worker turnover as a symptom of a lack of meaningful support. At New Hope Children's Hospital (Chapter 6) an effective senior administrator would have traced the middle management's lack of cohesiveness to the CEO's style of divide and conquer. At Thurston High School (Chapter 9) an effective principal would have related the teachers' and students' disconnections from their respective peers and the violence in the school to the lack of opportunities for students to become personally known by others.

Each of these diagnostic processes is anchored by a leader's insistence that presenting symptoms are signals about larger, underlying forces that threaten work on a primary task. Moreover, presenting symptoms are not proof that people have bad intentions, are unskilled or lazy, or are of limited capacity. Symptoms are understood as adaptive attempts gone awry rather than expressions of innate inadequacy (Waters & Lawrence 1993). Disturbed systems, like individuals, try as best they can to cope with difficult circumstances. At times they do so badly. Changing them involves looking for the healthy impulses that reside within maladaptive behaviors (Waters & Lawrence 1993). Dysfunctional patterns of group and intergroup behavior – for example, at Greenvale Residential Treatment Center (Chapter 7), in which staff members form small groups for support and cut themselves off from colleagues – offer information about members' underlying strivings, their longings for mastery and belonging. Attended to as such, problematic behaviors provide valuable clues about healthy desires rather than simply unhealthy practices.

Effective change leaders thus look not to rid themselves and their units of problematic individuals, as did so many of the leaders profiled in Part 2, but seek instead more complex solutions for underlying disturbances. It is natural, even inevitable, that leaders, along with their members, develop simplified stories that lead to simplified solutions, as in the Maple Hospital SU (Chapter 10), which sought to solve its problems by firing the nurse manager. Often, such solutions cast those leaders and their allies in a soft, blameless light and let the harsh glare of responsibility fall upon those more distant (and often less powerful), rather than examine the underlying relationships between the two. This reflects immature defenses. As Friedman (1985: 58) notes, "Anxious systems diagnose people instead of their relationships. Therefore, the amount of diagnosing of others going on is an indication of the amount of anxiety present in the system." Effective leaders contain anxiety by holding onto their explanatory stories lightly, enabling the possibility that other stories will emerge that will help to make sense of a variety of people's experiences and perspectives.

Ideally, leaders create diagnostic processes that invite others' participation. Members are asked about their experiences, perceptions, and behaviors (Alderfer 1980b; Levinson 1991). This information is offered back to members, who help make sense of the results, generating and evaluating hypotheses to explain them. Those explanations need to be sufficiently complicated, accounting for entire systems rather than seemingly problematic or disturbed individuals or groups. Using the interpretive stance (Shapiro & Carr 1991), effective leaders use own their feelings, perceptions, and experiences to identify underlying issues and processes and make them available for examination. When others follow their lead, sharing experiences from the perspectives of their own roles, system members develop a shared, nuanced understanding of the emotions, projections, and defenses that course beneath and shape their work. They develop shared pictures of the underlying plays they collude to stage. They develop shared insights about how they have collectively coped with stressful situations by creating disturbances that distracted them from the direct experience of anxiety, at some cost to their work with careseekers and with one another.

The diagnostic process is a crucial platform for organizational change. It can be the means by which leaders create a compelling case for transformational change. Such change requires certain conditions: significant business opportunities, committed leaders, and energized members (Weisbord 2004). The diagnostic process brings these together, making the case for change, displaying leaders' commitment, and energizing people by disrupting their denial or contentment, thus making them more available for change (Weisbord 2004). Effective leaders use the diagnostic process to get others to feel an appropriate sense of urgency. They use the process to move them toward the difficult and necessary work of interrupting status quos marked by casualties and losses that they are no longer willing to tolerate.

Engagement

Transformational change cannot occur without organization members engaging in understanding problems and designing and implementing solutions. Widespread participation in change processes is closely related to their success. Leaders must enable members to participate in meaningful ways. On one level, this entails framing change projects and supporting members with the resources necessary to complete those projects. On another level, it means encouraging members to create new patterns of relationships with one another and with careseekers.

Engaging members in transformational change is most effectively accomplished through the use of projects – concrete tasks that focus on particular areas of organizational functioning that, while discrete enough to be accomplished by small groups, have a wider real and symbolic impact on the larger system. Framed correctly, projects are vehicles by which members simultaneously solve problems and develop more functional patterns of working and relating. They allow for the interruption of dysfunctional status quos.

At Greenvale Residential Treatment Center (Chapter 7), for example, such a project might involve the creation of a new structure for treatment teams. Each residential house would have its own treatment team, a small group composed of several representatives from each department who over time would coalesce into a unit able to develop a coordinated approach to interacting with specific clients in accordance with their needs. This project would serve multiple aims simultaneously. It would create a better model for interdepartmental collaboration than that currently in play in the agency. It would fill the void left by the lack of an agency-wide sense of a therapeutic milieu. It would allow teams to develop and implement treatment plans for clients that reduce how they split and play members of different departments against one another. The creation of a new structure for treatment teams, supported by training and logistical solutions, would constitute a project by which dysfunctional processes are interrupted and replaced with more functional ones that better serve the agency's primary task.

Such projects – which might include the creation of a new process for patient flow into and through the Sudbury Hospital ER (Chapter 8), a violence prevention project at Thurston High School (Chapter 9), or a surgical identification process in the Maple Hospital SU (Chapter 10) – tap into members' desires to work more effectively and efficiently. They offer people the opportunity to solve problems in healthy ways. Such healthy striving typically exists among members but their shared defenses against anxiety have too often diverted such impulses into disturbing patterns of thought and action.

Effective leaders convene groups of people to work on useful change projects. In groups, people can solve complex organizational problems and at the same time form new and different working relationships crucial to the success of transformational change efforts. The composition of project groups is important. Ideally, they are composed of members who represent the various formal and informal groups that exist in the unit or organization more generally. Such "microcosm groups" (Alderfer & Smith 1982) inevitably contain relations between the various organizational and identity groups in the organization, which shape how people work together on their projects. Since these intergroup relations probably need to be altered to support significant organizational change, the use of microcosm groups enables those relations to be "re-presented," i.e., made available for examination, during the course of the project group.

The leader's task here is twofold. First, it involves helping project group members reflect on how their relations with one another "re-present" those between the external groups to which they belong. Second, it involves pressing project group members to shift how they perceive and work with one another, to the point that they shed the disturbing aspects of the intergroup relations extant in the larger system. This process enlarges project group members' capacities for reflecting on and altering disturbances in their relations with one another. It also holds the promise of altering intergroup relations in the larger system, as members emerge from their project groups and model for the larger community more functional ways to collaborate with those previously deemed unacceptably "other."

Leaders also need to help create the external conditions under which project groups are successful. At one level, this involves providing necessary resources, including appropriate personnel, financing, and opportunities for visibility. At another level, it involves helping members create and maintain appropriate boundaries. Change projects trigger anxiety inside and outside the project groups themselves. Project group members will experience pulls upon them by their own departments, functions, hierarchical levels, and other groups to retain the status quo, which, even if not entirely beneficial to those groups, is at least familiar. They will experience their own internal pulls as well – to withdraw from, undermine, or in other ways not fully engage in the project group. The leader needs to maintain boundaries impermeable enough to enable members to turn away from their external pulls and toward one another, yet permeable enough to enable members to remain sufficiently connected to their own groups to represent them properly. Project groups are small insurrections that need to be protected, particularly while their members struggle with their own impulses to lay down their arms.

Engaging the embedding organization in transformational change processes involves many of the steps of classic organizational change programs (Kotter 1996; Lewin 1951). The project groups are working on small experiments in the form of new programs, services, processes, and structures. Leaders need to ensure that the results of these experiments are communicated more broadly, either as small wins on which they can now build or as small failures from which much can be learned. Increasingly larger forums need to be created that enable unit and organization members to react to organizational diagnoses, the work of project groups, and evolving plans for systemic change. Leaders must ensure that meaningful opportunities for participation exist and are embraced as such.

Containment

People are understandably anxious about letting go of familiar ways of thinking and acting. They are anxious about having to create different kinds of working relationships. They are anxious about performing new tasks and roles that may require of them certain capabilities they are not sure they possess or can acquire. At a deeper level, they are anxious about the newly-uncertain meaning of their experiences. As Stapley (1996: 171) writes, "In developing a culture the members of an organization develop a structure of meaning. Any change is liable to undermine the very structure of meaning on which it has come to rely for its sense of continuity, consistency, and confirmation." The result, he notes, is grief. "If grieving is a response to loss of meaning, then it should be provoked by all situations of loss, including organizational change, where the ability to make sense of life is severely disrupted" (p. 173). Organization members engaged in a transformational change process experience loss, in ways small and large. Their work involves not simply engaging the substance of the change but finding ways to both mourn their losses and develop new frameworks of meaning.

Effective leaders understand the importance of enabling people to work through experiences of letting go of the familiar. These leaders make visible to others their own beliefs that the lack of discussion about loss, anxiety, and uncertainty related to significant organizational change is likely to undermine its ultimate effectiveness. They render familiar and predictable the stages of change, which involve as a matter of course the kinds of experiences – shock, denial, anger, sadness – common to the experience of death (Kubler-Ross 1997). Moreover, these leaders help create and authorize the settings (such as supervision, department meetings, and organizational forums) in which people's experiences of loss can be surfaced and validated in the course of their creating new work structures and frameworks of shared meaning.

Leaders must also make themselves personally available to others working through their experiences of change. Organization members need their leaders as temporary attachment figures to steady them during change processes (Byng-Hall 1998; Miller 1993; Stapley 1996). Significant change requires courage, as people move from familiar if maladaptive patterns to unfamiliar if healthier ones. Such courage is enabled by the steady presence of a secure base, a trusted other to whom one can turn for support at moments of unsteadiness, confusion, and uncertainty (Bowlby 1980). It is difficult for people to be fully self-reliant without the sense that such a secure base is available for them should the need arise (Kahn 2002). The secure base role "includes identifying dangers and conflicts and making sure that any necessary measures are taken. A sense of security comes from knowing that worrisome situations will be tackled; it is not based on being reassured while ignoring the dangers" (Byng-Hall 1998: 123). People may thus feel safe enough to explore their new circumstances, to move into and through uncertainty, and take the risks necessary to create new ways of working and relating. As Vaillant (1993: 326) writes, "We can all display more mature defenses if we feel that our dependency needs may be met."

In their role as temporary secure bases during change processes, effective leaders contain others' anxieties. They "serve as a container during the 'working through' of change, so as to tackle not only the overt problem but also the underlying difficulties" (Miller 1993: 234). Such difficulties are related to members' natural fear and uncertainty as they move away from familiar defenses against anxiety. Caregiving organization members instinctively look to their leaders to contain their anxieties: their dependency needs heightened by the uncertainties of transitions, they wish for their leaders to hold, on their behalf, their anxieties and help them reflect on their meanings. Leaders do this by listening to and validating others without judgment. They reflect on rather than react to others and their experiences. This enables others to develop coherent stories about why and how their emotions arose and they acted as they did (Byng-Hall 1998).

Leaders able to serve members in such ways maintain what Friedman (1985) refers to as a "non-anxious presence." He offers a useful metaphor with which to describe this term, in the context of discussing how effective clergy members help their congregations navigate difficult organizational transitions:

> Members of the clergy function as transformers in an electrical circuit. To the extent that we are anxious ourselves, then, when anxiety in the congregation permeates our being, it becomes potentiated and feeds back into the congregational family at a higher voltage. But to the extent that we can recognize and contain our own anxiety, then we function as step-down transformers, or perhaps circuit breakers. In that case, our presence, far from escalating emotional potential, actually serves to diminish its "zapping" effect.
>
> (Friedman 1985: 209)

"Non-anxious" leaders avoid being drawn into others' defensive responses and routines; they hold the optimistic expectation that others can manage, given enough time and space to process their experiences.

Creating capacity

Finally, caregiving organization leaders help members enlarge their capacities for containing and working through their own anxieties during change processes. As Roberts (1994d: 82) writes, "Since institutional defenses arise in response to the anxieties inherent in the work, dismantling defensive structures requires providing alternative structures to contain these anxieties." She identifies three such alternative structures: positive acknowledgement of others' work, such that members feel clearly recognized and valued; holding environments, small stable groups in which staff reflect together on their work and share some of the unacceptable feelings it arouses, with positive support from management; and mechanisms for inviting, considering, and implementing ideas for change from everyone in the system so they can join in problem-solving and feel a sense of contribution toward shared purpose. Each of these enables caregiving organization members to withstand, separately and together, both daily stress and the upheaval of significant change: they enable resilience. They inoculate members against daily stress and episodic distress. They also create safety nets, woven from networks of strong relationships, into which members may tumble when they feel dislocated by significant changes.

Networks of social support among unit and organization members are the primary means by which to enlarge their capacities for managing change and its attendant anxiety. Indeed, they are a primary means by which to replace immature with mature defenses more generally. "Social supports," notes Vaillant (1993: 109), "are often a superior alternative to defense mechanisms." Other people help alleviate anxiety and depression. He continues, noting that:

> Social support can give us permission to share our conflict, and more important, permission to express and thus to attenuate the associated affect. Social supports also provide a "safe house" where affects can be given expression while the conscience is held at bay. The rituals of a funeral service and of sitting shivah are examples of social supports as an antidote to unbearable anxiety and depression. Others share responsibility for the mourner's pain.
>
> (Vaillant 1993: 109)

The act of sharing responsibility – of reaching out to someone, taking them by the arm or helping them to their feet, staying close by while listening to what they have to say about an experience they have just gone through or witnessed, acknowledging one's own close or distant participation in that experience, figuring out together what to do to deal with its implications – is at once simple and profound. It may make all the difference, to individuals and to organizations: "Social supports facilitate mature defenses," writes Vaillant (1993: 131); "loneliness fosters immature defenses." Effective leaders ensure that no members will remain lonely, split off from the rest of the system, casualties lost in the march of change.

Holding authority

The ability of caregiving units and organizations to transform into increasingly mature systems is, in the final analysis, intimately related to their leaders' abilities to hold authority in certain ways. They must authorize themselves to lead others toward some preferred future. They must hold authority lightly, enabling others to meaningfully engage change on their own terms and assume responsibility. They must also hold authority with some courage, given the pulls on (and within) them to resort to familiar if flawed status quos.

Holding firmly

Leaders engaging significant organizational change must authorize themselves to lead. In practice this means that they take stands: they tell members that current practices must change, articulate the reasons why, and hold firmly to the belief that their units and organizations can and will change. These stands are, ideally, principled rather than simply opportunistic or political. They are anchored by leaders' valuing of careseekers and their needs. Leaders hold firmly to primary tasks. They base their arguments for change on the need to improve their work with careseekers, and they mean it. They drive themselves and others to design and implement changes that support those arguments.

In the course of making strong arguments for change, leaders differentiate themselves. Differentiation in the psychological sense refers to a person's capacity to define his or her goals and values apart from what Bowen (1978) referred to as "surrounding togetherness pressures." Systems are more likely to change when leaders define their goals and values according to primary tasks while trying to maintain a non-anxious presence within the system (Friedman 1985). Within systems undergoing significant transition there is great pressure upon members to huddle together beneath familiar frameworks. This is an anxious response to systemic change and leaders must step away from this response in order to define goals and values in terms unfamiliar, and threatening, to others. This can free them and others to develop a wide repertoire of responses to crisis. Yet if their units or organizations are overly anxious, swept up in social defenses, members are not likely to respond well: "Anxious systems are less likely to allow for differentiated leaders," writes Friedman (1985: 29), "while leaderless systems are more likely to be anxious." The only choice, then, is for leaders to stand clearly for what they believe and hope others follow as best they can.

Holding lightly

Leadership and followership are intimately related (Berg 1998). Leaders holding firmly to the need for rigorous change require followers who come to believe that need, and further, become convinced that they need to engage the change process. Transformational change, as noted earlier, occurs when system members participate widely and deeply in devising ways to move toward shared goals. With enough belief and enough sense of ownership, members will improvise new ways of working and relating. They will rewrite their own scripts, not simply follow those of their leaders. The leader's role here is to hold a clear vision on behalf of others. When leaders authorize themselves to do so, good followers can authorize themselves to make the articulated visions their own and to figure out how to make them real.

Effective leaders thus hold lightly to their formal authority. They understand that their authority is only on loan and may be withdrawn by followers who experience betrayal, abandonment, or the abuse of power. They also understand that system members will look to them, at times longingly and at other times angrily, during discomforting transitions. Leaders must hold their authority at those times but not so tightly that members cannot later regain their autonomy. As Miller (1993: 254) writes, "Leadership [needs to be] strong enough and resilient enough to contain the dislodged dependency, and at the same time sophisticated enough to relinquish it again as the new system [becomes] established." Leaders are temporary attachment figures during change processes. To the extent they focus on managing those attachments effectively rather than on using power (i.e., maintaining and enhancing status and control), they enable system members to retain autonomy and work on behalf of primary tasks.

Holding courageously

Leaders also require courage to stay the course of change in spite of internal and external pulls not to. Others will pull them toward the status quo. They will invoke traditional stories to justify familiar work patterns. Members will seduce leaders, offering themselves in myriad ways in return for the cessation of the leaders' quests for differentiation and change. They will question the leader's competence and vision, stage insurrections, broker treaties, all in the hope of forcing leaders to back away or be distracted from change efforts. They will nod, smile agreeably, and act as if they are behind the change when they are not. Effective leaders are aware of such responses. They are not surprised by them, understanding them for what they are: people's natural reactions to the threat and anxiety of moving from certain if flawed presents to uncertain futures. Even with such awareness, however, leaders need the courage to challenge others.

They need the courage to challenge themselves as well. As noted earlier, effective leaders understand that dysfunctional patterns of behavior in their organizations have something to do with *them*. Through acts of commission or omission leaders have implicitly colluded with others to create or leave in place such patterns. They need courage to acknowledge those collusions. In this respect, courage is the opposite of shame, which involves retreat, covering up, hiding, and self-protection. Courage requires openness, vulnerability, and direct engagement (Waters & Lawrence 1993). Effective change leaders work through their sense of shame rather than let it derail their efforts. They delve into, learn about, and forgive themselves for colluding with disturbing patterns of thought and action.

Finally, there is the courage that leaders and members alike display in creating truly caregiving systems, in which they join together within and across various boundaries to support primary caregivers in spite of all the pressures upon them not to. On the face of it, this seems like simply a reasonable prescription for a functioning organization, whose members work together well enough to meet their goals and the needs of those seeking their help. Beneath the surface, however, this is a radical agenda. Truly caregiving systems must confront, in ways simple and profound, the emotional life coursing beneath the daily performance of tasks. This requires courage.

It requires a love of the tasks that drew people to their work and their organizations. It requires commitments to others – to students, clients, patients, congregants – that trump commitments to defending oneself against anxiety and against difficult feelings that one did not plan on having. It requires, finally, holding fast in the struggle to care well for others.

Final reflections

In working with caregiving organizations I am invariably struck by their members' insistence that their particular organizations are unique, and uniquely irrational. They point to some dysfunctional or surreal set of circumstances that has been allowed to remain – some system, policy, or dynamic that clearly goes against what the organization is trying to accomplish – and insist that only in *their* organization could such a thing occur. This is true enough, in that specific events and people exist in one place and not another. It is also not true. Irrationality appears across caregiving organizations, rooted not simply in specific circumstances but in the very nature of the caregiving enterprise. As I have argued and illustrated throughout this book, caregiving organizations are shaken and bent by the nature of their work with careseekers, whose experiences of learning, growing, and healing contain powerful emotional as well as cognitive elements. Some organizations and their members live and work well with those elements, bending but not breaking, regaining enough of their shape to serve incoming waves of careseekers. Other organizations and their members bend to the point where something snaps; they become disturbed and are unable to retain their resilience in the face of the ongoing strain.

The difference between these organizations is often a matter of degree. Resilient organizations undergo periods of disturbance, just as disturbed organizations experience periods of resilience. What sends one organization toward one type of steady state – resilience or disturbance – rather than another seems to be the abilities of its leaders and members to retain some reflective capacity, to create some spaces in which they examine and develop insights about their experiences. When they are able to do that regularly they tend more toward resilience than disturbance. They are able to understand the essential nature of the caregiving organization, as a setting rife with possibilities for vibrant connections between caregivers and careseekers. With enough reflective space, organization members can examine their experiences with careseekers for the clues they offer about how to best meet those people's needs. They can take in, digest, and learn about others. Without such reflective space, it is difficult to interrupt the dysfunctional, disturbing patterns in which they find themselves, for they are unable to decipher those patterns and their implications for how they ought to work with careseekers. They are left to collude with and repeat those patterns, uninterrupted.

I use the holding image quite a lot in this book. It is metaphorical, of course. A leader or supervisor does not physically hold an anxious social worker or nurse in the way that a mother holds a startled infant. Yet the metaphor has its adult analogues. Adults hold one another in various ways: they hold their gazes, they hold them to their word or their task, they hold fast to promises made, they hold tightly to others' words for inspiration or guidance. Such phrases but hint at the importance of adults needing and providing support, particularly in times of anxiety. Unless such support exists – people hearing one another out, taking in one another, absorbing and containing their anxiety, validating their experiences, and developing insights together – caregiving organization members remain stuck with their anxiety. They will discharge it in often inappropriate ways, harmful to themselves, their work, their relations with others, and, ultimately, to those who seek their care. They will flail about and create casualties.

The real work of caregiving organization leaders and members alike is to halt processes that create casualties, either of caregivers or careseekers. Any system or process that routinely sacrifices others (staff or careseekers) is disturbed. It saps organizational resilience. Once that is recognized – and the signs are clear to those willing to look at them without prejudice – people must make choices. They must choose whether to go along with or interrupt the disturbing patterns. This is a difficult choice. The former is familiar, routine. The latter is unknown, uncertain, bound to raise anxiety and resistance. It is also the path toward a meaningful attempt to pursue, in good faith, the organization's primary task.

It is with this last point that I end this book. The primary task of any organization is its reason for existence. The primary task of a caregiving organization is, ideally, the meeting of the needs of those who seek its services, such as students, addicts, patients, congregants, or other types of client. When members and leaders hold fast to that task, in the way that sailors hold fast to the topmast in the midst of roiling seas, they create the possibility for conversations, interpretations, conflicts, and mutual engagements that are in careseekers' best interests. When they drop that task, in uncertainty or fear or anxiety, and rather than search for and pick it up again, substitute others in its place, they do a disservice to others, if not to themselves. Resilience is a matter of dropping to one's knees, alongside others, and looking for what has been dropped, and is then standing again, holding as tightly to the task of meeting others' needs as one can. Such is the reason that these organizations exist and is the saving grace for those who work within them.

References

Abram, J. (1996) *The Language of Winnicott*. Northvale, NJ: Jason Aronson, Inc.

Ainsworth, M. D. S. (1967) *Infancy in Uganda: Infant Care and the Growth of Attachment*. Baltimore, MD: Johns Hopkins Press.

Ainsworth, M. D. S. (1990) Some considerations regarding theory and assessment relevant to attachments beyond infancy, in M. T. Greenberg, D. Cicchetti and E. M. Cummings (eds) *Attachment in the Preschool Years*. Chicago: University of Chicago Press.

Alderfer, C. P. (1980a) Consulting to underbounded systems, in C. P. Alderfer and C. L. Cooper (eds) *Advances in Experiential Social Processes* 2, pp. 267–95. New York: Wiley.

Alderfer, C. P. (1980b) The methodology of organizational diagnosis, *Professional Psychology*, 11: 459–68.

Alderfer, C. P. (1987) An intergroup perspective on group dynamics, in J. Lorsch (ed.) *Handbook of Organizational Behavior*, pp. 190–222. Englewood Cliffs, NJ: Prentice-Hall.

Alderfer, C. P. and Smith, K. K. (1982) Studying intergroup relations embedded in organizations, *Administrative Science Quarterly*, 27(1): 35–66.

Balint, M. (1968) *The Basic Fault*. London: Tavistock Publications.

Baranowsky, A. B. (2002) The silencing response in clinical practice: on the road to dialogue, in C. R. Figley (ed.) *Treating Compassion Fatigue*, pp. 155–70. New York: Brunner-Routledge.

Bayes, M. and Newton, P. M. (1985) Women in authority: a sociopsychological analysis, in A. D. Colman and M. H. Geller (eds) *Group Relations Reader* 2, pp. 309–22. Washington: A.K. Rice Institute.

Beaton, R. D. and Murphy, S. A. (1995) Working with people in crisis: research implications, in C. R. Figley (ed.) *Compassion Fatigue*, pp. 1–20. Florence, KY: Brunner/Mazel.

Berg, D. N. (1998) Resurrecting the muse: followership in organizations, in E. Klein, F. Gabelnick and P. Herr (eds) *The Psychodynamics of Leadership*. Madison, CT: Psychosocial Press.

Bertalanffy, L. von (1950) An outline of general systems theory, *British Journal of the Philosophy of Science*, 1: 134–65.

Bion, W. R. (1961) *Experiences in Groups*. New York: Basic Books.

Bion, W. R. (1962) *Learning from Experience*. London: Heinemann.

Bowen, M. (1978) *Family Therapy in Clinical Practice*. New York: Jason Aronson.

Bowlby, J. (1980) *Attachment and Loss*, (vol. 3). New York: Basic Books.

Bowlby, J. (1988) *The Secure Base*. New York: Basic Books.

Braxton, E. T. (1995) Angry children, frightened staff: implications for training and staff development, *Residential Treatment for Children and Youth*, 13(1): 13–28.

Byng-Hall, J. (1998) *Rewriting Family Scripts*. New York: The Guilford Press.

Catherall, D. (1995) Preventing institutional secondary traumatic stress disorder, in C. R. Figley (ed.) *Compassion Fatigue*, pp. 232–48. Florence, KY: Brunner/Mazel.

Cherniss, C. (1980) *Staff Burnout*. Beverly Hills, CA: Sage.

Cohen, Y. (1984) Residential treatment as a holding environment, *Residential Group Care & Treatment*, 2(3): 33–43.

Dartington, A. (1994) Where angels, fear to tread: idealism, despondency and inhibition of thought in hospital nursing, in A. Obholzer and V. Z. Roberts (eds) *The Unconscious at Work*, pp. 101–9. London: Routledge.

Dutton, J. E. (2003) *Energize your Workplace*. San Francisco: Jossey-Bass.

Fairbairn, W. R. D. (1952) *Psycho-analytic Studies of the Personality*. London: Routledge & Kegan Paul.

Figley, C. R. (1995) Compassion fatigue as secondary traumatic stress disorder: an overview, in C. R. Figley (ed.) *Compassion Fatigue*, pp. 1–20. Florence, KY: Brunner/Mazel.

Fine, M. (1994) Chartering urban school reform, in M Fine (ed.) *Chartering Urban School Reform*, pp. 5–30. New York: Teachers College Press.

Freud, A. (1936) *The Ego and the Mechanisms of Defense*. New York: International Universities Press.

Freud, S. (1959) *Group Psychology and the Analysis of the Ego*, ed. J. Strachey. New York: W. W. Norton.

Freud, S. (1977) *Inhibitions, Symptoms and Anxiety*, ed. J. Strachey. New York: W. W. Norton.

Friedman, E. H. (1985) *Generation to Generation*. New York: The Guildford Press.

Frost, P. (2003) *Toxic Emotions at Work*. Boston, MA: Harvard Business School Press.

Gaylin, W. (1976) *Caring*. New York: Knopf.

Goffman, E. (1959) *The Presentation of Self in Everyday Life*. New York: Doubleday Anchor.

Gould, L. J. (1993) Contemporary perspectives on personal and organizational authority, in L. Hirschhorn and C. Barnett (eds) *The Psychodynamics of Organizations*. Philadelphia, PA: Temple University Press.

Guggenbuhl-Craig, A. (1971) *Power in the Helping Professions*. New York: Spring Publishers.

Gustafson, J. P. and Cooper, L. (1985) Collaboration in small groups, in A. D. Colman and M. H. Geller (eds) *Group Relations Reader 2*, pp. 139–50. Washington: A. K. Rice.

Halton, W. (1994) Some unconscious aspects of organizational life: contributions from psychoanalysis, in A. Ohbolzer and V. Z. Roberts (eds) *The Unconscious at Work*, pp. 11–18. London: Routledge.

Heard, D. (1982) Family systems and the attachment dynamic, *Journal of Family Therapy*, 4: 99–116.

Herman, J. (1997) *Trauma and Recovery*. New York: Basic Books.

Hinshelwood, R. D. (2001) *Thinking About Institutions*. London: Jessica Kingsley Publishers.

Hinshelwood, R. D. and Skogstad, W. (2000) The dynamics of healthcare institutions, in R. D. Hinshelwood and W. Skogstad (eds) *Observing Organizations*, pp. 3–16. London: Routledge.

Hirschhorn, L. (1988) *The Workplace Within*. Cambridge, MA: MIT Press.

Hirschhorn, L. (1997) *Reworking Authority*. Cambridge, MA: MIT Press.

Jacques, E. (1974) Social systems as a defense against persecutory and depressive anxiety, in G. Gibbrard, J. Hartmann and R. Mann (eds), *Analysis of Groups*. San Francisco: Jossey-Bass.

Josselson, R. (1992) *The Space Between Us*. San Francisco: Jossey-Bass.

Jourard, S. M. (1971) *Self-disclosure*. New York: Wiley.

Kahn, W. A. (1992) To be fully there: psychological presence at work, *Human Relations*, 45(4): 321–49.

Kahn, W. A. (1993) Caring for the caregivers: patterns of organizational caregiving, *Administrative Science Quarterly*, 38(4): 539–63.

Kahn, W. A. (1995) Organizational change and the provision of a secure base: lessons from the field, *Human Relations*, 48(5): 489–514.

Kahn, W. A. (1998) Relational systems at work, *Research in Organizational Behavior*, 20: 39–76.

Kahn, W. A. (2001) Holding environments at work, *Journal of Applied Behavioral Science*, 37(3): 260–79.

Kahn, W. A. (2002) Managing the paradox of self-reliance, *Organizational Dynamics*, 30(3): 239–56.

Kahn, W. A. (2003) The revelation of organizational trauma, *Journal of Applied Behavioral Science*, 39(4): 364–80.

Kahn, W. A. and Kram, K. E. (1994) Authority at work: internal models and their organizational consequences, *Academy of Management Review*, 19(1): 17–50.

Kahn, W. A., Cross, R. and Parker, A. (2003) Layers of diagnosis for planned relational change in organizations, *Journal of Applied Behavioral Science*, 39(3): 259–80.

Kaplan, H. I. and Sadock, B. J. (eds) (1989) *Comprehensive Textbook of Psychiatry*, 5th edn. Baltimore, MD: Williams & Wilkins.

Kets de Vries, M. F. R. and Miller, D. (1985) *The Neurotic Organization*. San Francisco: Jossey-Bass.

Klein, J. (1987) *Our Need for Others*. London: Tavistock Publications.

Klein, M. (1959) Our adult world and its roots in infancy, *Human Relations*, 12: 291–303.

Kohut, H. (1977) *The Restoration of the Self*. Madison, CT: International University Press.

Kotter, J. (1996) *Leading Change*. Boston, MA: Harvard Business School Press.

Kouzes, J. M. and Posner, B. Z. (2002) *The Leadership Challenge*, 3rd edn. San Francisco: Jossey-Bass.

Kozol, J. (1991) *Savage Inequalities*. New York: Crown Publishers.

Kubler-Ross, E. (1997) *On Death and Dying*. New York: Scribner.

Levinson, H. (1991) Diagnosing organizations systematically, in M. F. R. Kets de Vries *et al.* (eds) *Organizations on the Couch*. San Francisco: Jossey-Bass.

Lewin, K. (1951) *Field Theory in Social Science*. New York: Harper & Row.

Likert, R. (1967) *The Human Organization*. New York: McGraw-Hill.

Lyth, I. M. (1988) *Containing Anxiety in Institutions: Selected Essays*, vol. 1. London: Free Association Books.

Main, T. F. (1995) *The Ailment and other Psychoanalytic Essays*. London: Free Association Books.

Maslach, C. (1982) *Burnout: The Cost of Caring*. Englewood Cliffs, NJ: Prentice-Hall.

Mawson, C. (1994) Containing anxiety in work with damaged children, in A. Obholzer and V. Z. Roberts (eds) *The Unconscious at Work*, pp. 67–74. London: Routledge.

Mayeroff, M. (1971) *On Caring*. New York: Harper & Row.

McCollom, M. E. (1990) Reevaluating group development, in M. McCollom and J. Gillette (eds) *Groups in Context*, pp. 133–54. Reading, MA: Addison-Wesley.

Memmi, A. (1974) *Dependence*. Boston, MA: Beacon Press.

Miller, A. (1981) *The Drama of the Gifted Child*. New York: Basic Books.

Miller, E. (1993) *From Dependency to Autonomy*. London: Free Association Books.

Miller, E. and Gwynne, G. (1972) *A Life Apart*. London: Tavistock Publications.

Minuchin, S. (1974) *Families and Family Therapy*. Cambridge, MA: Harvard University Press.

Modell, A. (1976) The holding environment and the therapeutic action of psychoanalysis, *Journal of the American Psychoanalytic Association*, 24: 285–307.

Moylan, D. (1994) The dangers of contagion: projective identification processes in institutions, in A. Obholzer and V. Z. Roberts (eds) *The Unconscious at Work*, pp. 51–9. London: Routledge.

Myers, D. and Wee, D. F. (2002) Strategies for managing disaster mental health worker stress, in C. Figley (ed.) *Treating Compassion Fatigue*, pp. 181–212. New York: Brunner-Routledge.

Noddings, N. (1984) *Caring*. Berkeley, CA: University of California Press.

Obholzer, A. (1994) Managing social anxieties in public sector organizations, in A. Obholzer and V. Z. Roberts (eds) *The Unconscious at Work*, pp. 169–78. London: Routledge.

Obholzer, A. and Roberts, V. Z. (1994) The troublesome individual and the troubled institution, in A. Obholzer and V. Z. Roberts (eds) *The Unconscious at Work*, pp. 129–38. London: Routledge.

Oshry, B. (1999) *Leading Systems*. San Francisco: Berrett-Kohler.

Pines, A. M. and Aronson, W. (1988) *Career Burnout*. New York: Free Press.

Pines, A. M. and Maslach, C. (1978) Characteristics of staff burnout in mental health settings, *Hospital and Community Psychiatry*, 29: 233–7.

Powell, L. C. (1994) Interpreting social defenses: family group in an urban setting, in M. Fine (ed.) *Chartering Urban School Reform*, pp. 112–21. New York: Teachers College Press.

Powell, L. C. (1997) The achievement (k)not: whiteness and "black" underachievement, in M. Fine, L. C. Powell and L. M. Wong (eds) *Off White: Readings on Race, Power, and Society*. New York: Routledge.

Powell, L. C. and Barber, M. E. (2004) Savage inequalities indeed: irrationality and urban school reform, in S. Cytrynbaum and D. Noumair (eds) *Group Relations Reader 3*. Jupiter, FL: A. K. Rice Institute.

Rice, A. K. (1958) *Productivity and Social Organization*. London: Tavistock Publications.

Rice, A. K. (1963) *The Enterprise and its Environment*. London: Tavistock Publications.

Roberts, V. Z. (1994a) The self-assigned impossible task, in A. Obholzer and V. Z. Roberts (eds) *The Unconscious at Work*, pp. 110–18. London: Routledge.

Roberts, V. Z. (1994b) The organization of work, in A. Obholzer and V. Z. Roberts (eds) *The Unconscious at Work*, pp. 28–38. London: Routledge.

Roberts, V. Z. (1994c) Conflict and collaboration: managing intergroup relations, in A. Obholzer and V. Z. Roberts (eds) *The Unconscious at Work*, pp. 187–96. London: Routledge.

Roberts, V. Z. (1994d) Till death do us part: caring and uncaring in work with the elderly, in A. Obholzer and V. Z. Roberts (eds) *The Unconscious at Work*, pp. 77–83. London: Routledge.

Rogers, C. R. (1958) The characteristics of a helping relationship, *Personnel and Guidance Journal*, 37: 6–16.

Scarf, M. (1987) *Intimate Partners*. New York: Random House.

Scarf, M. (1995) *Intimate Worlds*. New York: Random House.

Schein, E. H. (1999) *Organizational Culture and Leadership*, 2nd edn. San Francisco: Jossey-Bass.

Schön, D. (1983) *The Reflective Practitioner*. New York: Basic Books.

Segal, H. (1981) *The Collected Works of Hanna Segal*. New York: Jason Aronson.

Seligman, M. (1998) *Learned Optimism*. New York: The Free Press.

Shapiro, E. R. and Carr, A. W. (1991) *Lost in Familiar Places*. New Haven, CT: Yale University Press.

Shay, J. (1994) *Achilles in Vietnam: Combat Trauma and the Undoing of Character*. New York: Simon & Schuster.

Skogstad, W. (2000) Working in a world of bodies, in R. D. Hinshelwood and W. Skogstad (eds) *Observing Organizations*, pp. 101–21. London: Routledge.

Smith, K. K. (1989) The movement of conflict in organizations: the joint dynamics of splitting and triangulation, *Administrative Science Quarterly*, 34(1): 1–20.

Smith, K. K. and Berg, D. N. (1987) *Paradoxes of Group Life*. San Francisco: Jossey-Bass.

Smith, K. K., Simmons, V. M. and Thames, T. B. (1989) "Fix the women": An intervention into an organizational conflict based on parallel process thinking, *Journal of Applied Behavioral Science*, 25(1): 11–29.

Stapley, L. F. (1996) *The Personality of the Organization*. London: Free Association Books.

Stokes, J. (1994) The unconscious at work in groups and teams: contributions from the work of Wilfred Bion, in A. Obholzer and V. Z. Roberts (eds) *The Unconscious at Work*, pp. 19–27. London: Routledge.

Trist, E. (1990) Culture as a psycho-social process, in E. Trist and H. Murray (eds) *The Social Engagement of Social Science*, vol. 1, pp. 539–45. London: Free Association Books.

Vaillant, G. (1993) *The Wisdom of the Ego*. Cambridge, MA: Harvard University Press.

Walsh, F. (1998) *Strengthening Family Resilience*. New York: The Guilford Press.

Waters, D. B. and Lawrence, E. C. (1993) *Competence, Courage and Change: An Approach to Family Therapy*. New York: W. W. Norton.

Weisbord, M. R. (2004) *Productive Workplaces*, 2nd edn. San Francisco: Jossey-Bass.

Weiss, R. S. (1982) Attachment in adult life, in C. Parkes and J. Stevenson-Hinde (eds) *The Place of Attachment in Human Behavior*, pp. 171–84. New York: Basic Books.

Wells, L. (1985) The group as a whole perspective and its theoretical roots, in A. D. Colman and M. H. Geller (eds) *Group Relations Reader* 2, pp. 109–26. Washington: A.K. Rice Institute.

Werner, E. E. (1993) Risk, resilience, and recovery: perspectives from the Kauai longitudinal study, *Development and Psychopathology*, 5: 503–15.

Werner, E. E. and Smith, R. S. (1992) *Overcoming the Odds: High Risk Children from Birth to Adulthood*. Ithaca, NY: Cornell University Press.

Winnicott, D. W. (1960) The theory of the parent infant relationship, *International Journal of Psychoanalysis*, 41: 585–95.

Winnicott, D. W. (1965) *The Maturational Processes and the Facilitating Environment*. New York: International University Press.

Zane, N. (1994) When "discipline problems" recede: democracy and intimacy in urban charters, in M. Fine (ed.) *Chartering Urban School Reform*, pp. 122–35. New York: Teachers College Press.

Index